Mental Health and Psychiatric Nursing

Third Edition

Margaret P. Benner, RN, PhD, CS

Psychiatric Consultation and Liaison Nurse
Visiting Nurse Association of Greater Philadelphia

Springhouse Corporation
Springhouse, Pennsylvania

Staff

Executive Director
Matthew Cahill

Editorial Director
June Norris

Art Director
John Hubbard

Managing Editor
David Moreau

Acquisitions Editors
Patricia Kardish Fischer, RN, BSN;
Louise Quinn

Clinical Consultant
Maryann Foley, RN, BSN

Editor
Carol Munson

Copy Editors
Cynthia Breuninger (manager),
Christine Cunniffe, Brenna Mayer,
Christina Ponczek, Pamela Wingrod

Designers
Arlene Putterman (associate art director), Lesley Weissman-Cook (book designer), Diane Armento-Feliz, Joseph Clark, Linda Franklin, Donald G. Knauss, Kaaren Mitchel, Matie Patterson, Mary Stangl

Typographers
Diane Paluba (manager), Joyce Rossi Biletz, Phyllis Marron, Valerie Rosenberger

Production Coordinator
Margaret Rastiello

Administrative Assistants
Beverly Lane, Mary Madden, Jeanne Napier

Manufacturing
Debbie Meiris (director), Pat Dorshaw (manager), Anna Brindisi, T.A. Landis

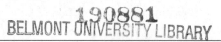

Printed in the United States of America.

SNMH3-011096

℞ A member of the Reed Elsevier plc group

Library of Congress Cataloging-in-Publication Data
Benner, Margaret P.
    Mental health and psyciatric nursing/Margaret P. Benner.—3rd ed.
    p. cm —(Springhouse notes)
    Includes bibliographical references and index.
    1. Psychiatric nursing.
    I. Benner, Margaret P. II.Title. III. Series.
    [DNLM: 1. Mental Disorders—nursing—outlines.
2. Psychiatric Nursing—outlines. WY 18.2B469m 1997]
RC440.B38 1997
610.73′68—dc20
DNLM/DLC   96-29146
ISBN 0-87434-862-5 (alk. paper)   CIP

Contents

Advisory Board and Reviewers iv
How to Use Springhouse Notes v

1. Roles and Functions of Psychiatric-Mental Health Nurses . . . 1
2. Conceptual Models of Psychiatric Care 11
3. Treatment Modalities and Roles of the Psychiatric Nurse . . 23
4. Stress and Psychophysiologic Disorders 33
5. Dying and Grieving 39
6. Alterations in Self-Concept 47
7. Anxiety and Related Behavioral Disorders 55
8. Mood Disorders 67
9. Suicide 80
10. Schizophrenic Disorders 88
11. Personality Disorders: Maladaptive Social Responses 100
12. Psychoactive Substance Abuse 108
13. Disorders Associated with Anger and Violence 123
14. Cognitive Impairment Disorders 141
15. Childhood and Adolescent Disorders 148

Appendices
A: Glossary 161
B: Answers to Study Questions 168
C: NANDA Taxonomy 176
D: *DSM-IV* Classification 179
E: Sexual and Sleep Disorders 193
Selected References 195
Index 196
StudySmart Disk . . . . inside back cover

Advisory Board and Reviewers

How to Use
Springhouse Notes

Springhouse Notes is a multi-volume study guide series developed especially for nursing students. Each volume provides essential course material in an outline format, enabling the student to review information efficiently.

Special features appear in every chapter to make information accessible and easy to remember. **Learning objectives** encourage the student to evaluate knowledge before and after study. **Chapter overview** highlights each chapter's major concepts. Within the outlined text, key points are highlighted in shaded blocks to facilitate a quick review of critical information. Key points may include cardinal signs and symptoms, current theories, important steps in a nursing procedure, critical assessment findings, crucial nursing interventions, or successful therapies and treatments. **Points to remember** summarize each chapter's major themes. **Study questions** then offer another opportunity to review material and assess knowledge gained before moving on to new information. **Critical thinking and application exercises** conclude each chapter, challenging students to expand on knowledge gained.

Other features appear throughout the book to facilitate learning: **Teaching tips** highlight key areas to address for patient teaching. **Clinical alerts** point out essential information on how to provide safe, effective care. **Decision trees** promote critical thinking. Difficult, frequently used, or sometimes misunderstood terms are indicated by SMALL CAPITAL LETTERS in the outline and defined in the glossary, Appendix A; answers to the study questions appear in Appendix B. Finally, a brand new Windows-based software program (see diskette on inside back cover) poses 100 multiple-choice questions in random or sequential order to assess your knowledge.

The Springhouse Notes volumes are designed as learning tools, not as primary information sources. When read conscientiously as a supplement to class attendance and textbook reading, Springhouse Notes can enhance understanding and help improve test scores and final grades.

Roles and Functions of Psychiatric-Mental Health Nurses

CHAPTER OVERVIEW

Since the late 1800s, trends and advancements in treatment, governmental acts, and changes in nursing standards and certification have shaped psychiatric-mental health nursing. As a result, contemporary psychiatric-mental health nurses have opportunities to work in a variety of roles (such as staff nurses, consultants, and researchers) and settings (such as hospitals, schools, clinics, and crises units). In any of these roles, the nurse's level of performance is determined by the nurse practice act and professional standards and by the nurse's education and experience, certification, practice setting, and personal initiative.

♦ I. Historical trends in psychiatric-mental health nursing care

A. 1880 to 1914
1. Provision of custodial care
2. Attention to the patient's physical needs
3. Medication administration
4. Assistance with hydrotherapy
5. Encouragement of the patient's participation in ward activities
6. Kindness toward and tolerance of the patient

B. 1915 to 1945
1. Expansion of the nursing care role through SOMATIC THERAPIES (nurses expected to provide emotional and physical care)
2. Recognition of the need for nurses with education and experience in psychiatry
3. Integration of psychiatric nursing into generic nursing curricula

C. 1946 to 1959
1. National Mental Health Act (1946), which authorized creation of the National Institute of Mental Health (NIMH) for research, training, and establishment of mental health centers
2. Availability of federal funding for collegiate nursing education and graduate degrees
3. Improvements in psychiatric nursing care standards
4. Use of tranquilizers, which shifted the focus of nursing care to therapeutic relationships and contributed to the trend toward deinstitutionalization
5. Development of psychiatric nursing theories as a basis for practice, including the work of Harry Stack Sullivan, whose theories helped define the nurse's role in MILIEU THERAPY
6. Mental Health Survey Act (1955), which created the Joint Commission on Mental Illness and Health to evaluate the needs and resources of mentally ill persons in the United States

D. 1960 to 1969
1. Shift in treatment from institutions to community mental health centers, in accordance with the Report of the Joint Commission (1961)
2. Community Mental Health Act (1963), which encouraged graduate education for nurses
3. Movement of psychiatric nurses into the community

    4. Expansion of the nurse's role to include promotion of mental health

E. 1970 to 1979
    1. Psychiatric nursing textbooks organized around the nursing process rather than the medical model
    2. Psychiatric nursing content integrated into nonpsychiatric courses
    3. Publication of *The Standards of Psychiatric-Mental Health Nursing Practice* (1973)
    4. Certification established by American Nurses Association (ANA) for psychiatric mental health nurse generalists (1973)
    5. President's Commission on Mental Health (1978), which emphasized the need for more community-based services and for increased mental health funding
    6. Certification established by ANA for psychiatric- mental health nurse specialists (1979)

F. 1980 to 1989
    1. Repeal of the Mental Health Systems Act (1981), cutting funds for psychological and social health services
    2. Withdrawal of federal funding from nursing education and from clinical training in psychiatric-mental health nursing
    3. Publication of revised *Standards of Psychiatric-Mental Health Nursing Practice* (1982)
    4. Creation of a national center for nursing research at the National Institutes of Health (1985)
    5. Creation of an NIMH task force on nursing (1987)
    6. Establishment of the National Mental Health Leadership Forum (1989)
    7. Scientific advances in psychobiology

G. 1990 to present
    1. "The decade of the brain"
    2. Integration of neuroscience into biopsychosocial psychiatric nursing practice
    3. Emphasis on sociocultural factors
    4. Refocus on care to balance high technology
    5. Revision of *Standards of Psychiatric-Mental Health Nursing Practice* (1993)
    6. Publication of *Psychopharmacology Guidelines for Psychiatric-Mental Health Nurses* by the ANA (1994)

◆ II. Psychiatric nursing roles

A. General information
    1. An interpersonal process used to promote, maintain, restore, or rehabilitate an individual's mental health

      2. A specialized area of nursing practice as defined by the ANA, that employs theories of human behavior as its science and "powerful use of self" as its art

      3. A skill that draws on psychosocial and biophysical sciences and on theories of personality and human behavior

      4. A profession that accepts individuals, families, groups, and communities as patients

      5. A core mental health discipline, as recognized by the NIMH

B. Current roles of psychiatric-mental health nurses

      1. Staff nurses

      2. Administrators

      3. Consultants

      4. Inservice educators

      5. Clinical practitioners

      6. Researchers

      7. Program evaluators

      8. Primary care providers

      9. Liaisons between the patient and other members of the health care delivery system

C. Psychiatric-mental health nursing functions

      1. General, as defined by the ANA

         a. Provide a therapeutic MILIEU

         b. Work to solve the patient's current problems

         c. Fulfill a surrogate parent role

         d. Use somatic therapies to alleviate the patient's health problems

         e. Educate consumers about factors (such as normal growth and development) that influence mental health

         f. Promote improved socioeconomic conditions

         g. Provide leadership to other personnel

         h. Conduct psychotherapy

         i. Engage in social and community mental health efforts

      2. PRIMARY PREVENTION

         a. Conduct health education

         b. Improve socioeconomic conditions

         c. Offer consumer education about normal growth and development

         d. Provide referrals before symptoms develop

         e. Support family members

         f. Engage in community and political activity

      3. SECONDARY PREVENTION

         a. Screen and evaluate patients promptly

         b. Visit the patient at home

         c. Provide emergency treatment

    d. Provide a therapeutic milieu
    e. Supervise patients on medication
    f. Prevent suicide
    g. Counsel on a time-limited basis
    h. Provide CRISIS INTERVENTION
    i. Conduct psychotherapy as an Advanced Practice Psychiatric-Mental Health Nurse
    j. Initiate community and organizational interventions (for example, assist with establishment of shelters for the homeless)
  4. TERTIARY PREVENTION
    a. Establish vocational training and rehabilitation programs
    b. Establish aftercare programs
    c. Recommend partial hospitalization, if appropriate
  5. Indirect activities
    a. Participate in inservice and continuing education
    b. Pursue nursing administration
    c. Supervise other personnel
    d. Engage in consultation and research
    e. Participate in legislative activities

D. Practice settings
  1. Psychiatric hospitals
  2. Community mental health centers
  3. General hospitals
  4. Community health agencies
  5. Outpatient clinics
  6. Homes
  7. Schools
  8. Prisons
  9. Health maintenance organizations
  10. Private practices
  11. Crisis units
  12. Industrial centers
  13. Residential facilities
  14. Partial hospitalization programs
  15. Day treatment centers
  16. Group homes

♦ III. Factors determining the performance level of psychiatric-mental health nurses

A. Nurse practice acts
  1. Regulate entry into the profession and define the legal limits of nursing practice (all states)
  2. Recognize the advanced practice of nurses (some states)

B. Education and experience
   1. Generalists—licensed registered nurses directly involved in mental health and psychiatric nursing; must meet the profession's standards of knowledge, experience, and quality of care; baccalaureate in nursing required by 1998
   2. Specialists—have graduate education, supervised clinical experience, and depth of knowledge, competence, and skill in their area of practice

C. Certification
   1. Requires a formal review process by the ANA
   2. Provides credentials for clinical practice, which certifies the nurse as either a generalist or a clinical specialist in adult or child psychiatric-mental health nursing.

D. Practice setting
   1. Organization's philosophy of mental illness, which helps shape the expectations of the patient and the nurse
   2. Administrative policies, which either foster or limit full use of nursing services

E. Personal initiative
   1. Willingness to act as an agent of change
   2. Knowledge of one's strengths and weaknesses
   3. Realization of clinical competence

F. Professional standards
   1. Developed by the ANA in 1982
   2. Define practice and performance (see *ANA standards of psychiatric and mental health nursing practice*)

POINTS TO REMEMBER

♦ Psychiatric nursing evolved in the late 19th and early 20th centuries.

♦ Psychiatric nursing uses interpersonal processes to promote, maintain, or restore mental health.

♦ Psychiatric nursing includes both direct and indirect care. Psychiatric nurses participate in primary, secondary, and tertiary levels of prevention.

♦ Many practice settings are available to psychiatric nurses.

ANA standards of psychiatric and mental health practice

Professional Practice Standards

Standard 1. Assessment
The psychiatric-mental health nurse collects client health data.

Standard 2. Diagnosis
The psychiatric-mental nurse analyzes the assessment data in determining diagnoses.

Standard 3. Outcome Identification
The psychiatric-mental health nurse identifies expected outcomes individualized to the client.

Standard 4. Planning
The psychiatric-mental health nurse develops a plan of care that prescribes interventions to attain expected outcomes.

Standard 5. Implementation
The psychiatric-mental health nurse implements the interventions identified in the plan of care.

Standard 5A. Counseling
The psychiatric-mental health nurse uses counseling interventions to assist clients in improving or regaining their previous coping abilities, fostering mental health, and preventing mental illness and disability.

Standard 5B. Milieu Therapy
The psychiatric-mental health nurse provides, structures, and maintains a therapeutic environment in collaboration with the client and other health care providers

Standard 5C. Self-Care Activities
The psychiatric-mental health nurse structures interventions around the client's activities of daily living to foster self-care and mental and physical well-being.

Standard 5D. Psychobiological Interventions
The psychiatric-mental health nurse uses knowledge of psychobiological interventions and applies clinical skills to restore the client's health and prevent further disability.

Standard 5E. Health Teaching
The psychiatric-mental health nurse, through health teaching, assists clients in achieving satisfying, productive, and healthy patterns of living.

Standard 5F. Case Management
The psychiatric-mental health nurse provides case management to coordinate comprehensive health services and ensure continuity of care.

Standard 5G. Health Promotion and Health Maintenance
The psychiatric-mental health nurse employs strategies and interventions to promote and maintain mental health and prevent mental illness.

Standard 5H. Psychotherapy
The certified specialist in psychiatric-mental health nursing uses individual, group, and family psychotherapy, child psychotherapy, and other therapeutic treatments to assist clients in fostering mental health, preventing mental illness and disability, and improving or regaining previous health status and functional abilities.

(continued)

ANA standards of psychiatric and mental health practice
(continued)

Professional Practice Standards *(continued)*

Standard 5I. Prescription of Pharmacologic Agents
The certified specialist uses prescription of pharmacologic agents in accordance with the state nurse practice act, to treat symptoms of psychiatric illness and improve functional health status.

Standard 5J. Consultation
The certified specialist provides consultation to health care providers and others to influence the plans of care for clients, and to enhance the abilities of others to provide psychiatric and mental health care and effect change in systems.

Standard 6. Evaluation
The psychiatric-mental nurse evaluates the client's progress in attaining expected outcomes.

Professional Performance Standards

Standard 1. Quality of Care
The psychiatric-mental health nurse systematically evaluates the quality of care and effectiveness of psychiatric-mental health nursing practice.

Standard 2. Performance Appraisal
The psychiatric-mental health nurse evaluates own psychiatric-mental health nursing practice in relation to professional practice standards and relevant statutes and regulations.

Standard 3. Education
The psychiatric-mental health nurse acquires and maintains current knowledge in nursing practice.

Standard 4. Collegiality
The psychiatric-mental health nurse contributes to the professional development of peers, colleagues, and others.

Standard 5. Ethics
The psychiatric-mental health nurse's decisions and actions on behalf of clients are determined in an ethical manner.

Standard 6. Collaboration
The psychiatric-mental health nurse collaborates with the client, significant others, and health care providers in providing care.

Standard 7. Research
The psychiatric-mental health nurse contributes to nursing and mental health through the use of research.

Standard 8. Resource Utilization
The psychiatric-mental health nurse considers factors related to safety, effectiveness, and cost in planning and delivering client care.

Standard 9. Interdisciplinary Collaboration
The nurse collaborates with other health care providers in assessing, planning, implementing, and evaluating programs and other mental health activities.

ANA standards of psychiatric and mental health practice
(continued)

Professional Performance Standards (continued)

Standard 10. Utilization of Community Health Systems*
The nurse participates with other members of the community in assessing, planning, implementing, and evaluating mental health services and community systems that include the promotion of the broad continuum of primary, secondary, and tertiary prevention of mental illness.
*Specific to clinical specialists with a master's degree in psychiatric or mental health nursing

Standard 11. Research
The nurse contributes to nursing and the mental health field through innovations in theory and practice and participation in research.

From *A Statement on Psychiatric-Mental Health Clinical Nursing Practice and Standards of Psychiatric-Mental Health Clinical Nursing Practice.* Washington, D.C.: American Nurses Association, 1994. Used with permission.

STUDY QUESTIONS

To evaluate your understanding of this chapter, answer the following questions in the space provided; then compare your responses with the correct answers in Appendix B, page 168.

1. What kinds of nursing care were delivered to mentally ill patients during the late 1800s and early 1900s?_____

2. What governmental legislation created the National Institute of Mental Health? _____

3. When did treatment for the mentally ill move from institutions to the community? _____

4. How does the ANA define the psychiatric nursing role? _____

_____

_____

5. What are the psychiatric nursing functions in primary prevention? _____

_____

_____

6. How do psychiatric nurse generalists differ from psychiatric nurse specialists? _____

_____

_____

CRITICAL THINKING AND APPLICATION EXERCISES

1. Develop a time line showing the trends in psychiatric nursing care from the late 1800's to the present. Highlight the major events.

2. Observe a nurse working in each of the following settings: a community mental health center and a psychiatric unit. Compare and contrast their roles and functions.

3. Obtain a copy of your state's nurse practice act. Prepare a class presentation that describes the act in detail.

Conceptual Models of Psychiatric Care

LEARNING OBJECTIVES

After studying this chapter, you should be able to:

♦ Discuss key aspects of the 11 theoretical models of personality and behavior.

♦ Identify each model's major theorists.

♦ Identify the underlying assumptions of each model.

♦ Describe the roles of the therapist and the patient within each model.

CHAPTER OVERVIEW

Mental health professionals often use conceptual models as a framework for clinical practice. Each model has certain assumptions and key ideas that form the basis for the therapeutic process. Throughout the process, the therapist or nurse has specific roles and functions.

♦ I. Behavioral model

A. General comments
   1. Rooted in psychology and neurophysiology, the behavioral model is associated with Pavlov, B.F. Skinner, and J. Wolpe
   2. The behavioral model regards symptoms as clusters of learned behaviors that persist because they are rewarded

B. Assumptions and key ideas
   1. Humans are complex animals
   2. The self is viewed as an individual's observable behavior
   3. Behavior is what an organism does
   4. People are shaped by elements in the environment
   5. The self is the structure of stimulus-response chains of habit
   6. Deviations occur when undesirable behavior is reinforced
   7. All behavior is learned

C. Therapeutic process
   1. The therapist's primary goal is to determine which patient behaviors should be changed and how
   2. The therapist helps effect change of undesirable behaviors
   3. Major treatments include DESENSITIZATION, OPERANT CONDITIONING, COUNTER-CONDITIONING, and TOKEN ECONOMY SYSTEM
   4. Behavior to be changed is reinforced
   5. Acknowledgment that change is an uncomfortable process

♦ II. Existential model

A. General comments
   1. This model was influenced by EXISTENTIALISM as found in the philosophical works of Sartre, Kierkegaard, and Heidegger
   2. Contemporary theorists include Frederick Perls, William Glasser, Albert Ellis, Carl Rogers, and R.D. Laing

B. Assumptions and key ideas
   1. Therapy focuses on the present
   2. Humans possess the freedom to realize their potential
   3. People act and are acted upon
   4. Behavior is mediated by self-awareness
   5. Self-awareness is modified by social interactions
   6. Deviations result when an individual is alienated from the self or the environment
   7. Lack of self-awareness prevents participation in authentic relationships

C. Therapeutic process
   1. Major treatments include GESTALT, RATIONAL-EMOTIVE, REALITY, and ENCOUNTER GROUP THERAPIES.

2. Therapy attempts to return the patient to an authentic awareness of being
3. Therapy focuses on the encounter between the patient and the therapist
4. The therapist and the patient are equal in their common humanity
5. The therapist acts as a guide, discouraging the patient's dependence on the therapist

◆ III. Medical model

A. General comments
   1. The medical model is based on the doctor-patient relationship
   2. The primary focus is on the diagnosis of mental illness
   3. The doctor uses the diagnosis to define treatment

B. Assumptions and key ideas
   1. Deviant behavior reflects a central nervous system disorder
   2. Environmental and social factors may precipitate illness or predispose a patient to it
   3. The doctor defines treatment to control symptoms and prescribes medication, surgery, and other modalities.
   4. Nurses direct the patient's care, supporting and coordinating holistic care in both acute and long-term management of mental illness
   5. Nurses play a key role in patient teaching and in monitoring medication

C. Therapeutic process
   1. The doctor examines the patient and diagnoses the illness, recording and classifying the diagnosis according to the American Psychiatric Association's *Diagnostic and Statistical Manual of Mental Disorders,* Fourth Edition, Revised *(DSM-IV)*
   2. The doctor prescribes treatment based on the diagnosis
   3. Therapy focuses on promoting the patient's trust, which fosters compliance with treatment
   4. The patient's role is that of a sick individual who must work to get well

◆ IV. Psychoanalytic model

A. General comments
   1. Sigmund Freud is the accepted father of this model
   2. Sexuality is a central concept in development
   3. Disruptive behavior in adults originates in earlier developmental stages
   4. Study of NEUROTIC BEHAVIOR led to this theory

B. Assumptions and key ideas
1. Psychic determinism governs human behavior
2. Unconscious processes occur in normal and abnormal mental functioning
3. Repressed feelings associated with conflict—and their release—are the focus of the theory
4. The topographic model of the mind includes the conscious, the preconscious, and the unconscious
5. The structural model of the mind includes the id, the ego, and the superego
6. Psychic energy derives from one's instincts or drives
7. Everyone uses defense mechanisms
8. Psychosexual development occurs in five stages
   a. Oral stage (0 to 18 months)
   b. Anal stage (18 months to age 3)
   c. Phallic stage (ages 3 to 5)
   d. Latency stage (age 5 to onset of puberty)
   e. Genital stage (pubescence to young adulthood)

C. Therapeutic process
1. The therapist may use FREE ASSOCIATION, dream analysis, hypnosis, and interpretation to help the patient recognize intrapsychic conflicts
2. The patient is motivated to work in therapy and develop insight into conflicts by TRANSFERENCE
3. Psychoanalysis can involve up to five meetings a week for several years

D. Other psychoanalytic theorists
1. Anna Freud expanded the area of child psychology
2. Melanie Klein developed play therapy in working with young children
3. Karen Horney related behavior to cultural and interpersonal factors
4. Freida Fromm-Reichman furthered the psychoanalytic theory of PSYCHOTIC BEHAVIOR
5. Karl Menninger developed levels of psychic dysfunction
6. Carl Jung added the concept of "collective unconscious"

♦ V. Developmental model

A. General comments
1. Erik Erikson expanded psychoanalytic models by including psychosocial and environmental influences
2. This model spans the total life cycle
3. Erikson identified eight stages of development (see *Erikson's eight stages of development*)

Erikson's eight stages of development

The table below highlights the eight stages of development identified by Erik Erikson.

DEVELOPMENTAL LEVEL	DEVELOPMENTAL TASKS	
Infancy	Trust	Mistrust
Toddler	Autonomy	Shame and doubt
Preschooler	Initiative	Guilt
School-age	Industry	Inferiority
Adolescent	Identity	Role confusion
Young adult	Intimacy	Isolation
Middle-aged adult	Generativity	Stagnation
Older adult	Integrity	Despair

B. Assumptions and key ideas
  1. Each stage of development includes critical tasks to be mastered and is considered an emotional crisis
  2. Mastery occurs more easily when chronologically appropriate
  3. Nonmastery of tasks inhibits movement to next stage
  4. Partial mastery of critical tasks leads to deficits in development
  5. Deficits progressively interfere with functioning
  6. Individual may have to return to earlier stage of development to resolve crisis

C. Therapeutic process
  1. Psychiatric patients often demonstrate developmental delays
  2. The therapist assesses degree of mastery of each stage up to chronological age
  3. The therapist addresses behavioral manifestations of developmental delays
  4. The therapist assists patient in mastering critical tasks

♦ **VI. Interpersonal model**

A. General comments
  1. The interpersonal model is associated with Harry Stack Sullivan

2. This model focuses on interactive aspects of behavior and development

B. Assumptions and key ideas
   1. Behavior is situationally produced and evolves within the context of interpersonal relationships
   2. Frequently motivated by anxiety, behavior is based on the drives for satisfaction and security
   3. Personality is an enduring pattern of interpersonal relationships
   4. People use SELECTIVE INATTENTION to defend against interpersonal anxiety
   5. The self-system resists change and consists of the "good me," the "bad me," and the "not me"
   6. Interpersonal development occurs in six phases
      a. Infancy (ages 1 to 2)
      b. Childhood (ages 2 to 6)
      c. Juvenile (ages 6 to 9)
      d. Preadolescence (ages 9 to 12)
      e. Early adolescence (ages 12 to 15)
      f. Late adolescence (ages 15 to 21)

C. Therapeutic process
   1. The therapist and the patient review the patient's life to explore progress through developmental stages
   2. Successful treatment depends on a healthy patient-therapist relationship
   3. Therapy involves reeducation; the therapist encourages the patient to learn more successful styles of relating
   4. The therapist's role is that of participant-observer

♦ VII. Cognitive model

A. General comments
   1. This model is most often associated with Jean Piaget and Aaron Beck.
   2. Cognitive functioning enables us to interpret the world around us and learn new skills
   3. The cognitive model describes how negative thinking can lead to development of symptoms of mental disorders

B. Assumptions and key ideas
   1. Piaget identified four major stages of cognitive development
      a. Sensorimotor
      b. Preoperational
      c. Concrete operational
      d. Formal operational

2. Movement through each stage depends on biological, intrapersonal, and interpersonal factors
3. Aaron Beck focused on how people view themselves and their world
   a. Dysfunctional behavior is related to misperceptions and misinterpretation of experiences
   b. Cognitive distortions result from inadequate view of self, negative misinterpretation of the present, and negative view of the future (cognitive triad)

C. Therapeutic process
   1. The model helps nurses assess learning capabilities prior to teaching
   2. The therapist assists patient to identify cognitive distortions
   3. The patient and therapist work together to correct cognitive triad
   4. This model is most effective for treating depression, anxiety, and panic disorders

◆ VIII. Social model

A. General comments
   1. The social model is associated with Gerald Caplan and Thomas Szasz
   2. This model considers the impact of the social environment on an individual

B. Assumptions and key ideas
   1. The self emerges through social interaction
   2. Deviance is culturally defined; it is not an illness
   3. Society labels "undesirables" as mentally ill
   4. Diagnosis and institutionalization are used to exert social control over deviants
   5. An individual takes responsibility for behavior by deciding whether or not to conform to social expectations
   6. Social situations, such as poverty or inadequate education, can predispose an individual to mental illness
   7. Crises can trigger deviant behavior

C. Therapeutic process
   1. Therapy promotes freedom of choice and community MENTAL HEALTH
   2. The patient defines the problem and initiates therapy
   3. The therapist (who may be professional or nonprofessional) collaborates with the patient to promote change

◆ IX. Stress-adaptation model

A. General comments
   1. The stress-adaptation model is associated with Hans Selye

General adaptation syndrome

The chart below describes the three stages of general adaptation syndrome and the physical and psychosocial changes that accompany each stage.

STAGE	PHYSICAL CHANGES	PSYCHOSOCIAL CHANGES
I. Alarm reaction (Body mobilizes its defenses and activates the "flight or fight" response)	• Release of norepinephrine and epinephrine: – vasoconstriction – increased blood pressure – increased rate and force of cardiac contraction • Increased hormone levels • Enlargement of adrenal cortex • Marked loss of body weight • Shrinkage of thymus, spleen, and lymph nodes • Irritation of gastric mucosa	• Increased level of alertness and anxiety • Task oriented • Defense oriented • Inefficient or maladaptive behavior
II. Resistance (Body adapts to stress within the person's capabilities)	• Readjustment of hormone levels • Reduced activity and size of cortex • Return of lymph nodes to normal size • Return of body weight to normal	• Coping mechanisms increased and intensified • Reliance on defense-oriented behavior
III. Exhaustion (Body loses its ability to resist stress because of depleted body resources)	• Decreased immune response – T cells suppressed – thymus atrophy • Depleted hormone production and adrenal glands • Weight loss • Lymphatic dysfunction • If exposure to stressor continues, cardiac failure, renal failure, or death may occur	• Defense-oriented behaviors exaggerated • Disorganized thinking and personality • Illusions and misperception of stimuli • Reduced contact with reality • If exposure to stressor continues, possible stupor or violence

    2. This model provides a framework for understanding how stress affects individuals and their responses

  B. Assumptions and key ideas

    1. Ability to adapt to stress leads to conflict resolution

    2. Inability to adapt effectively may result in physiologic or mental disorders and can lead to death

    3. General adaptation syndrome (GAS) occurs in three stages: alarm, resistance, and exhaustion.

    4. Physical and psychosocial changes can be associated with each GAS stage (see *General adaptation syndrome*)

C. Therapeutic process
1. Therapy focuses on assisting patients develop effective coping methods
2. The therapist helps patients identify and evaluate maladaptive and dysfunctional behaviors
3. The therapist facilitates problem solving and the use of adaptive behaviors
4. The therapist teaches stress management, problem solving, and relaxation techniques

◆ X. Nursing model

A. General comments
1. No universally accepted model exists; nursing theorists include H. Peplau (Interpersonal), D. Orem (Self-care), C. Roy (Adaptation), I. King (Systems), M. Rogers (Unitary Man), and Watson (Curative factors)
2. All nursing models incorporate a HOLISTIC approach
3. Nursing models focus on the patient's biological, psychological, and sociocultural needs and on nurse-patient responses

B. Assumptions and key ideas
1. Basic concepts include person, the environment, health, nurse, and nursing
2. Of primary importance is an individual's response to actual or potential health problems
3 Patient behavior results from a combination of predisposing factors and precipitating STRESSORS

C. Therapeutic process
1. The patient's needs are the focus of a therapeutic nurse-patient relationship
2. The patient and the nurse collaborate, with the nurse acting as patient advocate
3. The nurse intervenes at any point along the health-illness continuum
4. The nursing process guides care, and nursing care goals are based on nursing diagnoses established by the North American Nursing Diagnosis Association (NANDA) (see Appendix C, pages 176 to 178)
5. The nurse assists the patient in obtaining an optimum level of functioning.
6. Significant nursing functions include optimizing effective communication skills, coordinating health care, applying comfort measures to ease pain, helping the patient maximize capabilities, and teaching the patient

◆ XI. Biogenic model

A. General comments
 1. The biogenic model has been influenced by scientific investigations into the neuroanatomy and physiology of the brain
 2. The biogenic model examines biological factors that influence behavior
   a. Body types (ectomorph, endomorph, and mesomorph)
   b. Genetics (heredity)
   c. Neurotransmission
   d. Circadian rhythms
B. Assumptions and key ideas
 1. Body types correlate with personality traits and susceptibility to mental disorders
   a. Ectomorph—associated with schizophrenia
   b. Endomorph—linked with bipolar disorders
 2. Heredity and the environment interact, causing a genetic predisposition to mental disorders
 3. Mental disorders are often related to a deficiency in, an excess of, or an imbalance among NEUROTRANSMITTERS
 4. Circadian rhythms may affect physical and psychological well-being; this may explain the etiology of episodic or cyclical mental disorders
C. Therapeutic process
 1. Characteristics of therapy are similar to those of the medical model
 2. The biogenic model favors somatic treatments, such as PSYCHOSUR-GERY, electroconvulsive therapy, and medications

POINTS TO REMEMBER

◆ Assumptions about the development of personality and deviance vary by conceptual model.

◆ The functions and roles of the therapist and the patient differ within each conceptual model.

◆ Using a holistic approach, nursing models consider the patient's response to actual or potential health problems.

◆ The nurse-patient relationship is a collaboration, with the nurse acting as patient advocate.

STUDY QUESTIONS

To evaluate your understanding of this chapter, answer the following questions in the space provided; then compare your responses with the correct answers in Appendix B, page 168.

1. What key idea forms the basis of the behavioral model? _____

   _____

   _____

2. What are the roles of the therapist and the patient in the existential model?

   _____

   _____

3. What are the six phases of interpersonal development in the interpersonal model? _____

   _____

   _____

4. In the medical model, how is the diagnosis recorded and classified? _____

   _____

   _____

5. What is the focus of nursing models? _____

   _____

   _____

6. Who is the father of the psychoanalytic model? _____

   _____

   _____

7. What are the roles of the patient and the therapist in the social model?_____

   _____

   _____

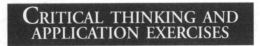

CRITICAL THINKING AND APPLICATION EXERCISES

1. Develop a table that compares and contrasts the major conceptual models used in psychiatric care.

2. Using Piaget's four stages of cognitive development, write examples for each stage.

3. Select a nursing model, and use it to describe an assigned patient.

CHAPTER

Treatment Modalities and Roles of the Psychiatric Nurse

LEARNING OBJECTIVES

After studying this chapter, you should be able to:

♦ Describe seven treatment modalities used with psychiatric patients.

♦ Discuss assumptions underlying crisis intervention, therapeutic environment, group approaches, family therapy, individual psychotherapy, and biological and cognitive behavioral therapies.

♦ Identify at least six curative factors for individual and group approaches.

♦ Compare and contrast techniques of intervention in various treatment approaches.

♦ Discuss the role of the nurse in each of the treatment modalities.

CHAPTER OVERVIEW

Various treatment modalities, each with specific assumptions and characteristics, can be used with psychiatric patients. Understanding the techniques for each is crucial to providing coordinated patient care. Although the nurse's role may vary with each modality, the primary role is that of patient advocate.

♦ I. Crisis intervention

A. Assumptions
1. Crisis is a temporary state that occurs when stress overwhelms an individual's usual coping mechanisms
2. Crisis is self-limiting, typically resolving within 6 weeks
3. Crisis intervention is an appropriate action for all nurses in all settings

B. Predisposing factors
1. Disastrous event
2. Threatened loss of a basic gratification
3. Failure to cope with stress
4. Perceived absence of situational support

C. Phases
1. Anxiety in response to a perceived threat or event
2. Disorganization with increased general anxiety
3. State of emergency with resolution or defeat
4. Breaking point

D. Types
1. Developmental-maturational crisis
2. Situational crisis
3. Victim crises

E. Characteristics of intervention
1. Increases the likelihood that a crisis will be positively resolved
2. Offers immediate help and reestablishes equilibrium
3. Restores the patient's precrisis level of functioning
4. Teaches the patient new ways of problem solving

F. Phases of intervention
1. Assess the nature of the crisis, its effect on the patient, and the patient's coping mechanisms and support systems
2. Begin planning: formulate dynamics, explore options, designate steps to arrive at solutions
3. Intervene through environmental manipulation, general support, or a generic or individual approach
   a. Environmental manipulation provides direct situational support or removes stress (such as arranging for someone to stay with the patient)
   b. General support reassures the patient that the health care professional understands and will help the patient (for example, by providing empathy)
   c. A generic approach uses a standard intervention for all individuals faced with the same crisis

      d. An individual approach uses interventions tailored to a particular patient

    4. Evaluate whether the crisis has been positively resolved

G. Techniques of intervention
1. Take an active, focal, and exploratory approach
2. Maintain the patient's present orientation
3. Guide intervention through its phases
4. Encourage expression of feelings and an awareness of the links among events, current feelings, and behavior
5. Persuade the patient to view the therapist as a helper

6. Promote and reinforce adaptive behavior
7. Do not attack the patient's defenses, which are the only means available for coping; doing so will only escalate the crisis
8. Increase the patient's self-esteem
9. Explore solutions to the problem causing the crisis

H. Alternative strategies
1. Telephone crisis counseling
2. Emergency department crisis counseling
3. Home visits
4. Family crisis counseling
5. Crisis group therapy

I. Role of the nurse
1. Assess the crisis
2. Offer individual crisis therapy
3. Organize crisis groups
4. Participate in disaster work
5. Use preventive intervention
6. Provide patient education

♦ **II. Therapeutic environment**

A. Assumptions
1. Scientific manipulation of the environment can change the patient's personality
2. Patients have strengths as well as conflict-free portions of their personalities, so they can constructively influence treatment
3. Successful treatment depends on therapeutic staff involvement at all levels
4. Human behavior can change in response to physical, interpersonal, and cultural environments

B. Characteristics of intervention
1. Focuses on a patient's interaction with the environment

2. Creates an atmosphere in which the patient can develop appropriate responses to individuals and situations
3. Is deliberately planned and structured to modify maladaptive responses
4. Promotes positive insights and responses

C. Treatment modalities
  1. MILIEU THERAPY
  2. Therapeutic community
  3. Community meeting
  4. Patient-team meeting
  5. Therapeutic recreation
  6. Occupational therapy
  7. Music and art therapy
  8. Horticulture therapy

D. Techniques of intervention
  1. Encourage, develop, and maintain communication between staff and patient
  2. Hold weekly staff meetings
  3. Set limits on and establish external controls over unacceptable behaviors
  4. Foster the patient's psychosocial skills
  5. Assess and implement individual treatment modalities
  6. Create a homelike atmosphere
  7. Focus treatment on action and problem solving

E. Role of the nurse
  1. Act as a role model primarily in inpatient settings
  2. Facilitate and oversee implementation of interventions
  3. Structure the patient's environment

♦ **III. Group approaches**

A. Assumptions
  1. Human beings are social animals that desire interaction with others
  2. Group therapy can alleviate intrapsychic distress or modify personality traits
  3. Therapeutic groups focus on interpersonal, cognitive, or behavioral changes
  4. Group dynamics can help modify behavior
  5. Groups offer a safe environment for sharing emotional experiences
  6. Essential components of group therapy were identified by I.D. Yalom in 1985

B. Stages of group development
  1. Initial: conflict issues are dependency and authority

2. Middle: conflict issues are intimacy, cooperation, and productivity
3. Final: conflict issues are disengagement and dissolution

C. Leadership styles
1. Democratic: encourages all members to participate in decision making
2. Autocratic: maintains control over decision making
3. Laissez-faire: relinquishes all control over decision making and provides little, if any, guidance or support

D. Membership roles in groups
1. Task roles: administrative and goal-oriented
2. Maintenance roles: enhance group interaction
3. Egocentric roles: express individual emotional needs

E. Yalom's curative factors in groups
1. Imparting information
2. Instillation of hope
3. Universality
4. Altruism
5. Corrective recapitulation of the primary family group member
6. Development of socializing techniques
7. Imitative behavior
8. Interpersonal learning
9. Group cohesiveness
10. Catharsis
11. Existential factors

F. Types of group leadership
1. Single therapist
2. Cotherapist
3. Leaderless

G. Types of group therapies
1. Psychotherapeutic groups
2. PSYCHODRAMA
3. Multiple-family group therapy

H. Types of therapeutic groups
1. Self-help groups
2. Remotivation and reeducation groups
3. Patient-government groups
4. Activity therapy groups
5. Patient teaching-education groups
6. Symptom-management groups
7. Stress-management groups

I. Role of the nurse in group approaches
  1. Group therapy must be conducted by a clinical specialist with a master's degree and a history of supervised clinical practice with groups
  2. Therapeutic groups can be conducted by all nurses in all settings

◆ IV. Family therapy

A. Assumptions
  1. Dysfunction in a patient usually originates in the family
  2. The family is the patient, and the focus is on family interaction
  3. The goal is to enable each family member to function independently

B. Models
  1. Structural therapy
  2. Strategic therapy
  3. Family systems therapy
  4. Multiple family therapy

C. Techniques and strategies
  1. Cotherapy
  2. Single therapist
  3. Network therapy
  4. Operational mourning
  5. Sculpting
  6. Role playing
  7. Paradoxical injunction

D. Role of the nurse
  1. A generalist nurse sees patients in a family context, recognizes functional and dysfunctional behavior patterns, then makes referrals
  2. A clinical specialist works as a family therapist and consultant

◆ V. Individual psychotherapy

A. Assumptions
  1. Therapy uses interpersonal relationships to effect positive changes in the patient's psychological well-being
  2. The need for help is typically expressed as a symptom
  3. The patient is anxious and usually depressed

B. Curative factors common to all theoretical approaches
  1. Common goal linking the therapist and the patient
  2. Mobilization of the patient's hope
  3. Anticipatory guidance
  4. Verbal communications
  5. Universality
  6. Emotional arousal
  7. Provision of new information

8. Insight into the problem's origin
9. Development of new problem-solving skills
10. Social learning experiences (such as new techniques for communicating with others)
11. Imitative behavior
12. Intense, confiding relationship

C. Types
  1. Crisis intervention
  2. Time-limited therapy
  3. Supportive therapy
  4. Long-term therapy

D. Role of the nurse
  1. A clinical specialist acts as a psychotherapist in therapy
  2. A generalist nurse acts as a supportive therapist by counseling and by maintaining the nurse-patient relationship

◆ VI. Cognitive behavioral therapy

A. Assumptions
  1. Maladaptive responses arise from cognitive distortions
  2. This theory applies learning theories to problems of living
  3. This theory views individual as decision maker
  4. This theory focuses on modifying thoughts, attitudes and beliefs, and behaviors
  5. The emphasis is on behavioral monitoring

B. Goals of treatment
  1. Increased activity
  2. Reduction of unwanted behavior
  3. Increased pleasure
  4. Enhanced social skills

C. Techniques of intervention
  1. Anxiety reduction
    a. Relaxation training
    b. Biofeedback
    c. Systematic desensitization
    d. Flooding
  2. Cognitive restructuring
    a. Monitoring thoughts and feelings
    b. Questioning the evidence
    c. Examining alternatives
    d. Decatastrophizing
    e. Reframing
    f. Thought stopping

    3. Learning new behavior
        a. Modeling
        b. Shaping
        c. Token economy
        d. Role playing
        e. Social skills training
        f. Aversion therapy
        g. Contingency contracting

D. Role of the nurse
    1. All nurses can use the theory in any setting to promote healthy coping responses
    2. The nurse assists the patient in developing new skills
    3. The nurse teaches cognitive behavioral techniques to others

♦ **VII. Biological therapies**

A. Assumptions
    1. Biological therapies follow a medical model
    2. They focus on symptoms, diagnoses, and prognoses

B. Types of biological treatments
    1. Psychotropic medications
    2. Electroconvulsive therapy
    3. NARCOTHERAPY
    4. PSYCHOSURGERY
    5. Niacin therapy
    6. Electrosleep therapy
    7. Nonconvulsive electrical stimulation therapy
    8. PHOTOTHERAPY
    9. HYDROTHERAPY

C. Role of the nurse
    1. Function as a patient advocate
    2. Educate the patient
    3. Administer medications
    4. Support the patient before, during, and after treatment
    5. Observe the patient for adverse reactions

POINTS TO REMEMBER

♦ Nurses must understand various treatment modalities to coordinate total care.
♦ The role of the nurse varies with each treatment modality.

◆ A nurse must act only in roles for which he or she is educationally and clinically prepared.

◆ The nurse's primary role is that of patient advocate.

STUDY QUESTIONS

To evaluate your understanding of this chapter, answer the following questions in the space provided; then compare your responses with the correct answers in Appendix B, page 169.

1. What is a crisis? How long does it usually last?_____

_____

_____

2. What are the major characteristics of crisis intervention? _____

_____

_____

3. What is the nurse's role in a therapeutic environment?_____

_____

_____

4. What are the three membership roles assumed in a group?_____

_____

_____

5. What is the focus of family therapy? _____

_____

_____

6. What are the roles of the clinical nurse specialist and the nurse generalist in individual psychotherapy? _____

_____

_____

7. What is the focus of biological therapies? _____

_____

_____

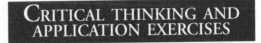

CRITICAL THINKING AND APPLICATION EXERCISES

1. Participate in a group therapy meeting. Identify the leadership style and the roles assumed by each member.

2. Observe a family therapy session. Prepare a class presentation describing the session, including techniques and strategies used.

3. Prepare a table of the major classes of psychotropic medications. List the actions, indications, possible adverse reactions, and nursing implications for each class.

CHAPTER

Stress and Psychophysiologic Disorders

LEARNING OBJECTIVES

After studying this chapter, you should be able to:

♦ Explain the concept of psychophysiologic disorders.

♦ Discuss the concept of stress.

♦ Name eight stress-related nonpsychiatric illnesses.

♦ Use the nursing process for patients with psychophysiologic disorders.

CHAPTER OVERVIEW

Based on the premise that mind and body are interrelated, a relationship exists between stress and psychophysiologic disorders. These nonpsychiatric medical conditions require a thorough assessment, including information about the patient's level of stress, coping abilities, belief systems, family dynamics, and support systems. Interventions focus on supporting the patient's efforts to reduce stress and on educating the patient about strategies to minimize and cope with stress.

◆ I. Stress

A. General information
   1. The mind and body are interrelated
   2. Stress is a state of imbalance within an organism brought about by an actual or perceived disparity between environmental demands (STRESSORS) and the organism's capacity to cope with them
   3. Stress manifests itself in various physiologic, emotional, and behavioral response patterns
   4. Any emotion, activity, or situation that requires a response can produce stress
   5. Psychophysiologic disorders are nonpsychiatric medical conditions caused by behavioral or psychological factors

B. Factors that influence stress response
   1. Intensity of the stimulus
   2. Duration of the stimulus
   3. Perception of control over the stimulus

C. Adaptation (physiologic responses) to stress
   1. General adaptation syndrome (GAS)
      a. Alarm
      b. Resistance
      c. Exhaustion
   2. Local adaptation syndrome
      a. Inflammatory, localized reaction to injury
      b. Reaction similar to GAS
   3. FIGHT-OR-FLIGHT RESPONSE
   4. Symptoms of stress
      a. Nervousness
      b. Inertia
      c. Insomnia
      d. Headache
      e. Dizziness
      f. Fainting
      g. Nightmares
      h. Hypertension
      i. GI distress

◆ II. Stress-related illness

A. Characteristics
   1. Any stressful experience may result in a psychophysiologic disorder
   2. Most patients do not consciously recognize stress
   3. Specific mind-body relationships are poorly understood by experts
   4. The primary behaviors observed are somatic symptoms

B. Predisposing factors
1. Endocrine activity affects personality
2. Some patients have a genetic tendency for particular psychological responses
3. Stressors produce physical and chemical changes in the body
4. Chronic stress damages the central nervous system
5. Most patients self-identify organs which may be affected by specific stressors
6. A relationship exists between immune system, stress, and certain psychophysiologic disorders.

C. Theories about psychological factors
1. Many clinical experts contend that a relationship exists between personality type and specific psychophysiologic disorders
2. Although specific psychological factors have been associated with certain physical conditions, no etiological theory has been proven
3. The patient's difficulty in dealing with feelings or in acknowledging their importance may contribute to a psychophysiologic disorder

D. Psychophysiologic disorders
1. Stress-related skin disorders may include allergy, eczema, hives, psoriasis, and acne
2. Stress-related respiratory system disorders may include breathlessness, hyperventilation, hay fever, asthma, sinusitis, emphysema, and bronchial spasms
3. Stress-related cardiovascular system disorders may include hypertension, migraine headaches, and coronary heart disease
4. Stress-related endocrine system disorders may include diabetes mellitus, gonadal dysfunction, and adrenal dysfunction
5. Stress-related musculoskeletal system disorders may include backache and muscle cramps
6. Stress-related GI system disorders may include colitis, gastritis, constipation, obesity, hyperacidity, duodenal ulcer, and anorexia
7. Stress-related genitourinary system disorders may include menstrual disturbances, impotence, and vaginismus
8. In extreme cases, death may result (research suggests that this represents the exhaustion phase of GAS)

♦ **III. Nursing assessment data**

A. Physical assessment

B. Psychosocial assessment

C. Measurement of stress level

D. Investigation of coping abilities

TEACHING TIPS
Patient with stress-related psychophysiologic disorder

Be sure to include the following points in your teaching plan for the patient.
- Causes of stress if known
- Measures to minimize stress before it becomes problematic
- Signs and symptoms of increasing stress
- Stress-management strategies
- Possible referrals for supportive therapy

  f. Behavior modification
  g. Yoga
  h. Exercise and stretching
  i. ATTITUDINAL RESTRUCTURING
  j. AUTOGENIC TRAINING
  k. Stress DESENSITIZATION
  l. Massage
  m. THERAPEUTIC TOUCH
  n. Psychotherapy
  o. Nutrition
  p. Laughter
  q. Play
  r. Music

◆ **VI. Evaluation**

  A. Base evaluation on identified patient care goals
  B. Do not interpret lack of goal achievement as failure

POINTS TO REMEMBER

◆ Stress manifests itself in various physiologic, emotional, and behavioral response patterns.

◆ General adaptation syndrome is a physiologic reaction to stress.

◆ Health care providers must not ignore the psychological needs of patients with physical symptoms.

◆ The nurse should offer support to patients with stress-related disorders.

◆ Nursing interventions can enhance the patient's ability to reduce and manage stress.

STUDY QUESTIONS

To evaluate your understanding of this chapter, answer the following questions in the space provided; then compare your responses with the correct answers in Appendix B, page 169.

1. What is stress? _____

_____

_____

2. Which three factors influence the stress response? _____

_____

_____

3. What are the three phases of general adaptation syndrome? _____

_____

_____

4. Which two types of diagnoses are used to identify stress and psychobiological disorders? _____

_____

_____

5. Which strategies can be used to manage stress? _____

_____

_____

CRITICAL THINKING AND APPLICATION EXERCISES

1. Interview a patient with a psychophysiologic disorder that determine how stress affects the condition. Describe measures that the patient uses to reduce stress.

2. Develop a patient instruction sheet for one stress-management strategy.

3. Choose two stress-management strategies, and try managing your own stress with each. Identify the advantages and disadvantages of each.

4. Develop a plan of care from admission through discharge for a patient with a psychophysiologic disorder. Be sure to include plans for follow-up and patient education.

CHAPTER

Dying and Grieving

LEARNING OBJECTIVES

After studying this chapter, you should be able to:

♦ Identify at least five emotions common to dying patients.

♦ Apply the nursing process for the dying patient and family.

♦ Name at least three behaviors associated with each of the following: uncomplicated, delayed, and distorted grief reactions.

♦ Apply the nursing process for patients experiencing uncomplicated grief reactions.

CHAPTER OVERVIEW

The concepts of dying and grieving are emotionally charged. Acceptance and support of the dying patient and the patient's family are crucial to facilitating the grieving process. If grief is delayed or distorted, the nurse must focus on helping the patient and the family work through their feelings.

♦ I. Dying

A. Theoretical perspectives
1. Natural death
   a. Occurs expectedly as a result of disease, thereby completing the life cycle
   b. Usually elicits an UNCOMPLICATED GRIEF REACTION from survivors because it is expected
2. Sudden death
   a. Occurs without warning, thereby terminating the life cycle
   b. Usually elicits a more prolonged or complicated grief reaction from survivors because it is unexpected

B. Stages of coping with anticipated dying
1. Denial
   a. Establishes a protective barrier
   b. Allows mobilization of other coping methods
   c. Should not be challenged by the nurse
   d. May manifest as an unwillingness to acknowledge symptoms, noncompliance, or refusal to discuss illness-related matters
2. Anger
   a. Commonly occurs after the patient perceives a loss of control
   b. Is usually directed toward others
3. Bargaining
   a. Constitutes an attempt to postpone the inevitable
   b. Commonly involves the dying person making a secret pact with God
4. Depression
5. Acceptance
   a. Wishes to be left alone
   b. Becomes less involved with others
   c. Appears devoid of all feelings
   d. Experiences a sense of closure

C. Common emotions of patients anticipating death
1. Loneliness
2. Sorrow
3. Fear of the unknown
4. Fear of dying alone
5. Loss of self-concept from altered body image
6. Regression and dependence
7. Loss of self-control
8. Fear of suffering and pain

D. Nursing assessment
1. Stage of coping
2. Emotional state

E. Diagnoses
　1. Related medical diagnoses
　　a. Dysthymic disorder
　　b. Major depressive disorder
　2. Related NANDA diagnoses
　　a. Ineffective individual coping
　　b. Anxiety
　　c. Hopelessness
　　d. Powerlessness

F. Nursing planning and implementation
　1. Outcomes
　　a. The patient and family members will accept that death will occur
　　b. The patient will participate in decision-making
　2. Interventions for the patient and family
　　a. Assist the patient in living more fully and comfortably
　　b. Help the family support the patient
　　c. Assist the patient and family members accept death
　3. Nursing interventions for the patient

**CLINICAL
ALERT**

　　a. Maintain a secure, caring atmosphere
　　b. Accept and support the patient's denial as a necessary COPING
　　　MECHANISM; confronting or attacking the patient's denial would
　　　exacerbate the patient's stress
　　c. Encourage the patient to participate in decisions that affect the
　　　patient's life
　　d. Understand the patient's anger
　　e. Encourage the patient to articulate needs and feelings
　　f. Help the patient schedule daily routines to include satisfying ac-
　　　tivities
　　g. Assist the patient in reviewing the past
　4. Nursing interventions for the family
　　a. Encourage the family to communicate openly with the patient
　　b. Recommend that family members help the patient complete un-
　　　finished business (making a will; settling financial affairs)
　　c. Reassure the patient and family that anger, depression, guilt, and
　　　a sense of loss are normal stages of grieving
　　d. Encourage family members to express their feelings about the pa-
　　　tient's anticipated death
　　e. Help family members adapt to changes in roles or lifestyles
　　f. Enlist family members in caring for the patient
　　g. Provide education to assist with death, dying and grieving (See
　　　Patient's family, page 42)

TEACHING TIPS
Patient's family

Be sure to include the following topics in your teaching plan for the family of a patient who is dying.
- Need for some patient control in the decision-making process
- Open communication among all involved
- Adaptation to role and lifestyle changes
- Expression and acknowledgment of feelings of all involved
- Available supports
- Coping strategies
- Stages of grieving

---

5. Evaluation
   a. Note whether the patient and family move toward acceptance of death
   b. Document evidence of maladaptive responses

♦ II. Grieving

A. Definitions
   1. Subjective response to the loss of a significant person or object
   2. Universal reaction that affects all aspects of one's life
   3. Emotion that typically impairs the ability to function
   4. Syndrome that usually has a predictable cause and effect

B. Types of grieving
   1. Uncomplicated grief reactions
      a. Shock and disbelief
      b. Heightened awareness
         (1) Intense and conflicting emotions, such as sadness and anger
         (2) Self-destructive behavior
         (3) Preoccupation with and yearning for the lost person
         (4) Guilt over perceived omissions
         (5) Acute symptoms of grief lasting 4 to 8 weeks
         (6) Disorganization of personality as hope of reunion is surrendered
      c. Reorganization, letting go, resolution
         (1) Detachment
         (2) Withdrawal
         (3) Investment of energy in new objects or people
         (4) Loss of future orientation
         (5) Painful review of memories
         (6) Process that typically lasts up to 1 year

2. Delayed grief reaction
   a. Persistent absence of emotions
   b. Maladaptive response that can occur in any phase of the grieving process; anniversary day of loss may trigger underlying emotions
3. Distorted grief reactions
   a. Excessive activity with no sense of loss
   b. Physical symptoms like those of the deceased person
   c. Psychophysiologic illness
   d. Progressive social isolation
   e. Extreme hostility
   f. Wooden and formal conduct
   g. Clinical depression
   h. Activities detrimental to one's social and economic good
   i. Euphoria

C. Manifestations of grieving
   1. Somatic distress
      a. Waves of distress lasting from 20 to 60 minutes
      b. Sighs and deep breathing when discussing grief
      c. Lack of strength
      d. Loss of appetite and sense of taste
      e. Tightness in throat
      f. Choking sensation accompanied by shortness of breath
   2. Preoccupation with image of the deceased person, characterized by:
      a. Daydreaming
      b. Mistaking others for the deceased person
      c. Becoming oblivious to surroundings
      d. Feeling a sense of unreality
      e. Fearing insanity
   3. Guilt
   4. Hostility
   5. Personality disorganization
      a. Loss of self-esteem
      b. Despair
      c. Transient HALLUCINATIONS
      d. Overwhelming feelings of loneliness, fear, and helplessness

D. Nursing assessment
   1. Stage of coping
   2. Emotional state

E. Diagnoses
   1. Related medical diagnoses
      a. Dysthymic disorder
      b. Major depressive disorder
   2. Related NANDA diagnoses

      a. Anxiety
      b. Ineffective individual coping
      c. Anticipatory grieving
      d. Hopelessness
      e. Powerlessness
      f. Spiritual distress

F. Nursing planning and implementation
  1. Outcomes
    a. The patient and family will successfully progress through the stages of grieving
    b. The patient will verbalize needs openly
  2. Interventions for uncomplicated grief reactions
    a. Be aware of own personal feelings about and reactions to death.
    b. Support a dying patient who is grieving

CLINICAL ALERT

      (1) Establish rapport and build trust
      (2) Provide ANTICIPATORY GUIDANCE by helping the patient prepare for death and its consequences for the patient's family; preparation helps promote feelings of control over the situation
      (3) Encourage patient to express feelings candidly
      (4) Discourage patient from lingering in one stage of grieving or from using activities to avoid grieving
      (5) Provide patient with opportunities to release tension and guilt
      (6) Promote an adequate balance of rest, sleep, and activity
      (7) Discourage use of daytime sedatives and tranquilizers
      (8) Discourage dependence on staff members or others
      (9) Encourage patient to interact with others and to plan for the future
      (10)Mobilize the patient's support systems
    c. Support the family
      (1) Communicate news of the patient's death to the family as a group, in a private setting
      (2 Respect the family's religious and cultural beliefs and practices
      (3) Permit outward expression of grief
      (4) Listen attentively, and express sympathy
  3. Interventions for delayed grief
    a. Help patient identify underlying emotions associated with loss
    b. Help patient progress through the stages of normal grieving
  4. Interventions for distorted grief
    a. Set goals according to the patient's needs (for instance, promote independence in a patient who has become overly dependent)
    b. Direct interventions toward specific behaviors (for instance, focus on personal hygiene if a patient's withdrawn behavior leads the patient to neglect cleanliness)

G. Evaluation
   1. Note the patient's progression through the stages of grieving
   2. Document evidence of or changes in maladaptive emotional responses

POINTS TO REMEMBER

♦ The nurse should not challenge denial as an initial coping mechanism.

♦ Grief is a universal response to loss. Uncomplicated grief reaction usually lasts about 1 year.

♦ The anniversary of a loss may trigger a delayed grief reaction.

♦ General nursing care goals for uncomplicated grief reactions should support the grieving process.

STUDY QUESTIONS

To evaluate your understanding of this chapter, answer the following questions in the space provided; then compare your responses with the correct answers in Appendix B, pages 169 and 170.

1. What are the five stages of coping with anticipated dying? _____

   _____

   _____

2. What is the focus of nursing care for the dying patient and family? _____

   _____

   _____

3. What are the three phases of uncomplicated grief?_____

   _____

   _____

4. Which symptoms are important in evaluating a grieving patient?_____

   _____

   _____

5. How should a nurse manage a patient who is experiencing a distorted grief reaction?_____

_____

_____

CRITICAL THINKING AND APPLICATION EXERCISES

1. Prepare a class discussion on the five stages of coping with anticipated dying. Role play, with other students, situations associated with each stage.

2. Develop a table comparing uncomplicated, delayed and distorted grief reactions.

3. Care for a patient who is dying. Prepare a patient-specific plan of care, including any needs for follow-up with the family.

4. Attend a bereavement support group meeting. Prepare an oral presentation describing what you observed, the issues discussed, and the methods suggested for dealing with them.

CHAPTER

6

Alterations in Self-Concept

LEARNING OBJECTIVES

After studying this chapter, you should be able to:

♦ Define self-concept.

♦ Describe three behaviors associated with alterations in self-concept.

♦ Formulate individual nursing diagnoses for patients experiencing alterations in self-concept.

♦ Develop a nursing care plan, including outcomes and interventions, for meeting the needs of patients experiencing alterations in self-concept.

CHAPTER OVERVIEW

Self-concept, a broad term that includes body image, identity, roles, self-esteem, and self-ideals, provides the basis for one's personality. Certain behaviors are associated with an altered self-concept and may be diagnosed medically as dissociative disorders. Nursing care focuses on assessing these behaviors and on intervening to promote the characteristics of a healthy personality.

♦ I. Self-concept

A. Definitions
   1. All notions, beliefs, and convictions that constitute a person's self-knowledge and that, if positive, allow an individual to function effectively
   2. A determinant of a person's relationships with others
   3. A frame of reference by which each person interacts with the world
   4. The consequence, in part, of experiences with significant others

B. Components
   1. BODY IMAGE
      a. Attitude toward one's body, which usually mirrors self-concept
      b. Sum of conscious and unconscious attitudes, continually modified by one's perceptions and experiences
      c. Significant influence on self-esteem and role perception
   2. IDENTITY
      a. Awareness of oneself
      b. Consequence of self-observation and judgment
      c. Synthesis of self-representations into an organized whole
      d. Consciousness of oneself as an individual
      e. Concept that emerges in adolescence
      f. Ego identity
         (1) Recognition of the self as separate from others
         (2) Acceptance of one's sexuality
         (3) Compatibility among other aspects of self
         (4) Congruence between self-regard and societal regard
         (5) Awareness of relationships among past, present, and future
         (6) Realistic self-goals
      g. Object of maturational, cultural, and physiologic stressors
   3. Roles
      a. Consist of socially expected behavior associated with one's function within the societal group
      b. Provide a way to test identity
      c. Enhance self-esteem when they are congruent with self-ideals
      d. Lead to role disturbances when conflicts emerge between independent and dependent functioning
      e. Produce role strain from stress associated with role expectations
      f. Lead to role conflict when a person is subjected to simultaneous contradictory expectations or when an individual's or society's expectations of role behavior are incongruent
      g. Can result in role ambiguity when knowledge about specific role expectations is limited
      h. May produce role overload when the individual is faced with an overly complex set of roles

4. SELF-ESTEEM
   a. Individual's sense of self-worth
   b. Beliefs that originate in childhood and that are modified throughout life
   c. Internalization of the reactions of others; anxiety occurs when the self is threatened
   d. High self-esteem: prerequisite to SELF-ACTUALIZATION
   e. Low self-esteem: factor in poorly developed interpersonal relationships
5. Self-ideals
   a. Individual's perception of how to behave, based on personal standards and societal norms
   b. Standards influenced by abilities, cultural factors, ambitions, desire to succeed and avoid failure, anxiety, and inferiority
   c. Prerequisite for mental health: congruency between self-ideals and self-concept

C. Characteristics of a healthy personality
   1. Positive and accurate body image
   2. Realistic self-ideal
   3. Positive self-concept
   4. High self-esteem
   5. Clear sense of identity
   6. Openness to others
   7. Satisfaction in life roles

◆ II. Altered self-concept

A. Nursing assessment of behaviors
   1. Low self-esteem
      a. Self-derision and criticism
      b. Minimization of one's ability
      c. Guilt and worry
      d. Physical manifestations (such as substance abuse or psychosomatic illness)
      e. Ambivalence or procrastination
      f. Denial of pleasure to oneself
      g. Disturbed interpersonal relationships
      h. Withdrawal from reality
      i. Destructive behavior (toward self or others)
   2. Identity confusion
      a. Lack of sense of continuity between past and present
      b. High degree of anxiety
      c. Fluctuations in feelings about self
      d. Uncertainty about self-characteristics

e. Withdrawal from reality
f. Exaggerated sense of self-importance
3. DEPERSONALIZATION
a. Inability to distinguish between internal and external stimuli
b. Difficulty distinguishing self from others
c. Feelings that the body has an unreal quality
d. Estrangement
e. Confusion about sexuality
f. Absence of emotion
g. Loss of spontaneity
h. Withdrawal
i. Disturbed perceptions of time and space
j. Impaired judgment and thinking
k. Loss of impulse control
l. Inability to derive sense of accomplishment

B. Diagnoses
1. *DSM-IV* medical diagnoses
a. Dissociative identify disorder
b. Dissociative fugue
c. Dissociative amnesia
d. Depersonalization disorder
2. Primary NANDA diagnostic categories
a. Altered thought process
b. Anxiety
c. Body image disturbance
d. Personal identity disturbance
e. Altered role performance
f. Self-esteem disturbance
g. Social isolation

C. Nursing planning and implementation
1. Requirements
a. The patient's active participation in planning and implementation of treatment
b. The patient's readiness for growth
c. Clear and explicit goals
d. Emphasis on strengths rather than the pathologic condition
e. Use of problem-solving techniques
f. Clear focus on the present
2. General outcomes
a. The patient will attain maximum self-realization and self-acceptance
b. The patient will demonstrate increased confidence and sense of self-worth

TEACHING TIPS
Patient with an altered self-concept

Be sure to include the following topics in your teaching plan for the patient with an altered self-concept.
• Possible etiology
• Specific measures to expand self-awareness, encourage self- exploration, and foster self-evaluation
• Identification of conflict and appropriate coping mechanisms
• Realistic planning and goal setting
• Positive reinforcement for goal achievement

CLINICAL ALERT

3. General nursing interventions
  a. To expand self-awareness
    (1) Accept the patient unconditionally; acceptance is essential for establishing trust and fostering a positive environment
    (2) Listen attentively
    (3) Encourage patient to discuss thoughts and feelings
    (4) Respond nonjudgmentally
    (5) Convey the expectation that the patient is capable of self-help
    (6) Identify patient's ego strengths
    (7) Confirm patient's identity
    (8) Reduce patient's anxiety level
    (9) Set limits on appropriate behavior
    (10) Assist with personal hygiene
    (11) Provide activities that can be easily accomplished
    (12) Increase the number and complexity of activities gradually
  b. To encourage self-exploration
    (1) Help patient accept positive and negative thoughts and emotions
    (2) Help patient identify strengths, weaknesses, and self-criticisms
    (3) Have patient describe a self-ideal
    (4) Help patient describe how he or she relates to others
    (5) Respond with empathy
    (6) Teach patient to recognize conflict and maladaptive coping (see *Patient with an altered self-concept,* for more information)
  c. To foster self-evaluation
    (1) Help patient identify relevant stressors, unrealistic goals, faulty perceptions, strengths, and maladaptive responses
    (2) Explore coping resources

(3) Use such techniques as SUPPORTIVE CONFRONTATION, ROLE CLARIFICATION, and PSYCHODRAMA

d. To help formulate a realistic plan of action

(1) Mutually identify adaptive coping responses

(2) Encourage patient to formulate self-goals and to try new behaviors

(3) Discuss the consequences of each goal

(4) Use such techniques as ROLE REVERSAL, ROLE MODELING, ROLE PLAYING and VISUALIZATION

CLINICAL ALERT

|

e. To assist in goal achievement

(1) Provide opportunities for patient to experience success; success reinforces positive feelings

(2) Reinforce healthy aspects of patient's coping skills

(3) Help identify and obtain needed resources

(4) Facilitate peer interactions and organize group activities

(5) Allow time to change

(6) Provide support and positive reinforcement

4. Evaluation

a. Note patient's ability to identify stressors

b. Document use of adaptive coping responses

◆ III. Dissociative disorders: amnesia; fugue; depersonalization disorders

A. Description

1. Triggered by severe psychosocial stress

2. Manifested by repression of or dissociation from anxiety-laden experiences, conflicts, aspects of self, or traumatic experiences

3. Shown by separation of portions of ego from total personality

B. Nursing assessment

1. Denial

2. Ego-splitting

3. Altered mental functions

4. Preoccupation with somatic symptoms

5. Amnesia

6. Dissociative identity disorder

C. Nursing interventions

1. Promote the patient's self-actualization

2. Encourage greater self-understanding

3. Assess readiness for growth

4. Identify realistic short-term goals

5. Encourage exploration of feelings

6. Focus on the patient, not on symptoms

Points to Remember

◆ A healthy personality is characterized by a positive and accurate body image, realistic ideals, a positive self-concept, high self-esteem, a clear sense of identity, and openness toward others.

◆ Behaviors associated with altered self-concept are varied but usually reflect low self-esteem, identity confusion, depersonalization, disturbed body image, and negative or delinquent identity.

◆ The patient must actively participate in treatment.

◆ Nursing interventions must focus on assisting the patient in problem solving.

Study Questions

To evaluate your understanding of this chapter, answer the following questions in the space provided; then compare your responses with the correct answers in Appendix B, page 170.

1. What are the five components of self-concept? _____

_____

_____

2. What are the three categories of behavior commonly associated with an altered self-concept? _____

_____

_____

3. What are the primary outcomes of the nurse when dealing with a patient who is experiencing an alteration in self-concept? _____

_____

_____

4. How can the nurse intervene to assist the patient with self-evaluation? _____

_____

_____

CRITICAL THINKING AND APPLICATION EXERCISES

1. Using the five components of self-concept, assess a patient's self-concept. Then analyze the patient's personality using the characteristics of a healthy personality.

2. Read about the diagnostic criteria for dissociative disorders in *DSM-IV*.

3. Prepare a class demonstration using role play, role reversal, and role modeling to illustrate behaviors that either foster or inhibit self-concept.

Anxiety and Related Behavioral Disorders

LEARNING OBJECTIVES

After studying this chapter, you should be able to:

♦ Name five characteristics of anxiety.

♦ Describe physiologic, behavioral, cognitive, and affective responses to anxiety.

♦ Develop nursing care outcomes and interventions for a patient with anxiety.

♦ Develop nursing care outcomes and intervention for patients with anxiety disorders.

CHAPTER OVERVIEW

Anxiety can be constructive or destructive. Mild anxiety enhances learning while moderate to severe levels of anxiety can interfere with a patient's ability to cope and function. Anxiety is manifested by physiologic, behavioral, cognitive, and affective responses. Nursing care for the patient with an anxiety disorder focuses on identifying maladaptive behaviors, assessing the patient, and helping the patient develop and use appropriate coping strategies.

◆ I. Anxiety

A. Characteristics
   1. Consequence of and behavioral response to stress, changes, or threats to one's SELF-CONCEPT
   2. Uneasiness caused by conflicts and frustrations that tax one's coping skills
   3. State of unexplained discomfort
   4. Source of energy that can be used constructively or destructively
   5. Nonspecific feeling of dread accompanied by symptoms of physiologic stress

B. Theories on the origin of anxiety
   1. Psychoanalytic view (Freud)
      a. Primary anxiety, a state of trauma and tension first produced by external causes, originates during birth
      b. Subsequent anxiety is the emotional conflict between the primitive impulses of the ID and the regulatory function of the SUPEREGO
   2. Interpersonal view (Sullivan)
      a. Anxiety originates in the early bond between mother and child
      b. The condition is related to fear of disapproval
      c. Developmental trauma leads to specific vulnerabilities and anxiety
      d. In later life, anxiety arises when the person perceives unfavorable responses from others
      e. Anger commonly results from a mild or moderate level of anxiety
   3. Cognitive-behavioral view
      a. Anxiety occurs when a threat or danger is perceived
      b. Behaviorists view anxiety as a learned maladaptive response to stress
   4. Neurobiological view
      a. Anxiety results from interaction with cortisol arousal and activation of the autonomic nervous system
      b. Cortical arousal occurs when fearful events stimulate the limbic systems
         (1) Limbic system assists in mediating internal and external environmental clues
         (2) Limbic system can affect major biochemicals (for example— serotonin, norepinephrine, and gamma-aminobutyric acid)

C. Levels of anxiety
   1. Mild
      a. Heightens alertness
      b. Widens perceptual field
      c. Enhances learning

2. Moderate
   a. Limits one's focus to immediate concerns
   b. Narrows perceptual field
   c. Causes selective inattention
3. Severe
   a. Greatly reduces perceptual field
   b. Focuses one's attention on details of immediate concern
   c. Directs behavior toward getting relief
   d. Causes one to seek guidance from others in order to focus on areas beyond the immediate concern
4. Panic
   a. Distorts perceptions
   b. Severely impairs rational thought
   c. Diminishes ability to focus, even with direction from others
   d. Increases motor activity
   e. Decreases ability to relate to others

D. Precipitating stressors
   1. May be positive or negative
   2. Can have physiologic, psychological, or environmental origins
   3. May be perceived subjectively
   4. Can arise from threats to biological integrity
   5. Can arise from threats to self-esteem
      a. Unmet expectations
      b. Unfulfilled needs for status and prestige
      c. Anticipated disapproval
      d. Inability to gain recognition from others
      e. Guilt

E. Nursing assessment
   1. Physiologic responses to anxiety
      a. Cardiovascular
         (1) Palpitations
         (2) Tachycardia
         (3) Increased or decreased blood pressure
         (4) Faintness
      b. Respiratory
         (1) Rapid, shallow breathing
         (2) Shortness of breath or gasping
         (3) Chest pressure
         (4) Lump in throat or choking sensation
      c. Neuromuscular
         (1) Increased reflexes
         (2) Eyelid twitching
         (3) Insomnia

        (4) Fidgeting or pacing
        (5) Generalized weakness
        (6) Tremors or trembling
        (7) Lack of coordination
    d. Gastrointestinal
        (1) Loss of appetite or revulsion toward food
        (2) Abdominal discomfort or pain
        (3) Nausea
        (4) Heartburn
        (5) Diarrhea
    e. Genitourinary
        (1) Sudden urge to urinate
        (2) Frequent urination
    f. Integumentary
        (1) Flushing or pallor
        (2) Sweating
        (3) Itching
        (4) Hot and cold spells
2. Behavioral responses to anxiety
    a. Restlessness
    b. Physical tension
    c. Startle reaction
    d. Rapid speech
    e. Interpersonal withdrawal
    f. Avoidance
3. Cognitive responses to anxiety
    a. Impaired attention
    b. Inadequate concentration
    c. Preoccupation
    d. Forgetfulness
    e. Blocking of thoughts
    f. Confusion
    g. Loss of objectivity
4. Affective responses to anxiety
    a. Edginess
    b. Impatience
    c. Uneasiness and tension
    d. FEAR
    e. Jumpiness
5. Coping strategies
    a. Task-oriented
        (1) Attack behavior: destructive if aggressive, or constructive if self-assertive

    (2) Physical or emotional withdrawal: destructive if it results in isolation

    (3) Compromise: usually constructive

  b. Ego-oriented

    (1) Unconscious defense mechanisms (such as denial or intellectualization) used to protect self when task-oriented strategies are unsuccessful

    (2) Detrimental defense mechanisms that result in ego disintegration if used to extreme

F. Diagnoses

  1. *DSM-IV* medical diagnoses

    a. Cardiovascular and respiratory disorders

    b. Endocrine disorders

    c. Neurologic disorders

    d. Substance-related intoxications

  2. NANDA diagnoses

    a. Anxiety

    b. Ineffective individual coping

    c. Fear

G. Nursing planning and implementation

  1. Outcomes

    a. The patient will demonstrate the ability to tolerate mild anxiety and show how to use that ability consciously and constructively

    b. The patient will engage in problem-solving

  2. General interventions

    a. Identify the patient's anxiety level and its overall effect

    b. Determine whether the patient's DEFENSE MECHANISMS are constructive or destructive

  3. Interventions for moderate anxiety

    a. Help the patient recognize anxiety and underlying feelings

    b. Design an individual teaching plan to help the patient cope with anxiety and to increase the patient's knowledge of stressors, coping mechanisms, and responses to anxiety

    c. Explore alternate coping strategies

    d. Promote relaxation

-INICAL ALERT

  4. Interventions for severe and panic anxiety levels

    a. Stay with the patient

    b. Remain calm, and assess own personal anxiety level; approaching the patient calmly and unemotionally reduces the risk of further stressing the patient's already high anxiety level

-INICAL ALERT

    c. Reduce stimuli

    d. Use short, simple sentences; patient's ability to focus and to relate to others is diminished

e. Administer medications, as needed
f. Help channel the patient's energy constructively
g. Encourage the patient to eat nutritious foods
h. Suggest activities to promote sleep at bedtime

H. Evaluation
1. Periodically judge the adequacy, effectiveness, appropriateness, efficiency, and flexibility of nursing goals and actions
2. Regularly evaluate personal strengths, limitations, and anxiety level

♦ II. Anxiety disorders

A. General characteristics of disturbed coping patterns
1. Inability to make choices
2. Internal conflict beyond conscious control
3. Repetition of thoughts and actions
4. State of sustained imbalance
5. ALIENATION or a feeling that thoughts and feelings are unrelated
6. Stress caused by EGO-DYSTONIC BEHAVIORS
7. Secondary gain (for example, getting increased attention from others as a result of being ill)
8. Manifestations of ritualistic, avoidant, clinging, distancing, and overly dramatic behaviors
9. Somatic symptoms that have no physical basis
10. Episodic amnesia
11. Multiple personalities
12. Underlying anxiety

B. Diagnoses
1. Related *DSM-IV* medical diagnoses
   a. Acute stress disorder
   b. Agoraphobia without panic attacks
   c. Generalized anxiety disorder
   d. Obsessive-compulsive disorder
   e. Panic disorder with agoraphobia
   f. Panic disorder without agoraphobia
   g. Post-traumatic stress disorder
   h. Social phobia
   i. Specific phobia
2. Related NANDA diagnoses
   a. Impaired adjustment
   b. Anxiety
   c. Ineffective individual coping
   d. Fear
   e. Powerlessness

  f. Disturbed self-esteem

  g. Social isolation

C. Nursing planning and implementation

 1. General outcomes for behavioral disorders associated with anxiety

  a. The patient will express anxious feelings as they occur

  b. The patient will identify methods of coping with anxiety without avoidance; ritualistic, or somatic behavior

  c. The patient will identify feelings as well as realistic strengths and weaknesses

  d. The patient will identify contributions to maladaptive behavior pattern

  e. The patient will identify ways of meeting personal needs

 2. General nursing interventions

  a. Administer and monitor antianxiety medications

  b. Help patient identify maladaptive behaviors

  c. Assist patient in developing coping strategies

  d. Teach relaxation strategies

D. Evaluation

 1. Use identified patient care goals as a basis for evaluation

 2. Identify reasons for nonachievement of goals

 3. List outcomes expected by the nurse and the patient

◆ III. Anxiety disorder: Generalized anxiety state

A. Description

 1. Generalized, persistent anxiety; usually only mildly incapacitating

 2. Symptoms unrelated to any other mental disorder; can persist for 1 month

 3. Minimum patient age for diagnosis: 18 years; median age at onset: 25 years

 4. Depression as a major disabling adverse effect

 5. Possible suicide attempts

B. Nursing assessment

 1. Motor (muscle) tension

  a. Fidgeting

  b. Easy startle reflex

  c. Muscle twitching

  d. Trembling

  e. Strained expression

  f. Fatigue

  g. Inability to relax

 2. Autonomic hyperactivity

  a. Sweating

  b. Flushing or pallor

      c. Elevated pulse and respiratory rate

      d. Cold or clammy hands

      e. Diarrhea

      f. Frequent urination

      g. Pounding heart

      h. Upset stomach

      i. Light-headedness

      j. Dizziness

      k. Hot or cold spells

      l. Tingling of hands or feet

   3. Apprehension

      a. Worry

      b. Anxiety

      c. Repetitive thoughts

      d. Fears of grave misfortune or death

   4. Vigilance and scanning

      a. Excessive attention to surroundings

      b. Hypersensitivity

      c. Distractibility

      d. Inability to concentrate

      e. Impatience

      f. Irritability

C. Nursing interventions

   1. Observe for signs of mounting anxiety, and take direct measures to moderate it

   2. Teach the patient to detect anxiety by making thoughtful observations

   3. Do not validate or encourage the patient's use of destructive coping mechanisms

   4. Discuss options for meeting the patient's needs

   5. Negotiate a contract to work on goals

   6. Alter the environment to reduce the anxiety or to meet the patient's needs

♦ IV. Anxiety disorder: Phobias

A. Description

   1. Intense, irrational fear of an external object, activity, or situation

   2. Fear that persists even though the patient recognizes its irrationality

   3. Resistance to insight-oriented therapies

B. Nursing assessment

   1. Persistent fear of specific places or things

   2. Displacement and SYMBOLIZATION

   3. Disruption in social or work life

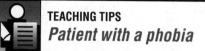

TEACHING TIPS
Patient with a phobia

Be sure to include the following topics in your teaching plan for the patient with a phobia.
• Identification (if possible) of object or situation causing anxiety
• Identification of coping mechanisms, resources and personal strengths
• Need for participation in desensitization therapy
• Relaxation techniques
• Ways to channel energy and relieve stress
• Reinforcement of positive coping mechanisms

4. Panic when confronted with the feared object

C. Nursing interventions
   1. Assist in desensitizing the patient
   2. Demonstrate progressive relaxation techniques
   3. Suggest that the patient substitute an alternate behavior
   4. Demonstrate healthier ways of coping; provide patient teaching (see *Patient with a phobia*)

◆ **V. Anxiety disorder: Obsessive-compulsive disorder**

A. Description
   1. Acute attacks, commonly triggered by stressful incidents
   2. Behaviors substituted for relating to others
   3. Distress

B. Nursing assessment
   1. Repetitive thoughts that the patient cannot control or exclude from consciousness
   2. Recurring, irresistible impulses to perform an action
   3. Defense mechanisms, such as isolation, UNDOING REACTION FORMATION, and MAGICAL THINKING

CLINICAL ALERT

C. Nursing interventions
   1. Do not set direct limits; patient is unable to control impulses
   2. Carefully weigh any interference with compulsive rituals
   3. Maintain a calm environment
   4. Remain sympathetic
   5. Avoid judging the patient
   6. Make reasonable requests for the patient to change
   7. Explain the reasons for change
   8. Engage in a constructive activity
   9. Reinforce nonritualistic behavior while encouraging the patient's efforts to explore the meaning and purpose of behaviors

10. Allow time for calming rituals (such as pacing) to show their effectiveness in reducing anxiety
11. Desensitize the patient toward feared objects or situations
12. Teach relaxation techniques

♦ VI. Anxiety disorder: Post-traumatic stress disorder

A. Description
   1. Stressors related to actual experiences; usually traceable to experiencing or witnessing a traumatic event
   2. Person responds to the event with intense fear, helplessness, or horror
   3. Ordinary coping behaviors ineffective
   4. Acute, chronic, or delayed reactions
   5. Likelihood of drug and alcohol use

B. Nursing assessment
   1. Flashbacks
   2. Dreams
   3. Nightmares
   4. Detachment
   5. Emotional numbness
   6. Hyperalertness
   7. Social isolation
   8. Chronic tension
   9. Labile affective responses
   10. Anxiety
   11. Guilt
   12. Anger
   13. Poor impulse control

CLINICAL ALERT

C. Nursing interventions
   1. Provide for patient safety; patient's ineffective coping coupled with the intensity of the reaction and poor impulse control increases the patient's risk of injury
   2. Encourage the patient to explore the meaning of the event
   3. Assist the patient with problem solving
   4. Teach relaxation techniques
   5. Encourage patient to join support groups

♦ VII. Somatoform and other disorders

A. Description
   1. Symptoms that carry a symbolic meaning
   2. Frequent remissions and exacerbations

B. Nursing assessment
   1. Physical symptoms without evidence of organic cause

2. Absence of psychological symptoms
3. Inability to resist distraction

C. Nursing interventions
1. Rule out any organic problems
2. Be aware of personal responses to the patient
3. Remember that the patient does not intentionally produce symptoms
4. Avoid reinforcing the symptoms
5. Assess the symbolic meaning of symptoms
6. Encourage the patient to express underlying anxiety
7. Increase the patient's self-esteem
8. Set limits for the patient
9. Teach relaxation techniques

POINTS TO REMEMBER

♦ Individuals exhibit physiologic, behavioral, cognitive, and affective responses to anxiety.

♦ Mild anxiety enhances learning.

♦ For moderate anxiety, the overall outcome is for the patient to develop the capacity to tolerate and use anxiety consciously and constructively.

♦ Patients who experience behavioral disorders associated with anxiety exhibit specific disturbed coping patterns.

♦ The nursing intervention goals for patients with disordered behaviors must be realistic.

♦ Nursing interventions should include helping the patient learn how to cope with anxiety-laden experiences.

♦ The nurse must monitor personal anxiety level.

STUDY QUESTIONS

To evaluate your understanding of this chapter, answer the following questions in the space provided; then compare your responses with the correct answers in Appendix B, page 170.

1. What are the six affective responses to anxiety? _____

_____

_____

2. What is the most important nursing intervention for dealing with a patient experiencing panic?_____

_____

_____

3. What is the minimum age for a patient to be diagnosed with generalized anxiety state? _____

_____

_____

4. What the key sign of a patient with a phobia? _____

_____

_____

5. What are the key signs and symptoms a nurse will notice when assessing a patient with an obsessive-compulsive disorder? _____

_____

_____

6. How should a nurse intervene when dealing with a patient experiencing a post-traumatic stress disorder?_____

_____

_____

7. What is the focus of nursing interventions for a patient with a dissociative disorder?_____

_____

_____

CRITICAL THINKING AND APPLICATION EXERCISES

1. Develop a table comparing the four theories on the origins of anxiety.

2. Ask a classmate to describe what happens when feeling anxious. Identify the responses as physiologic, behavioral, cognitive, or affective.

3. Research the therapies for treating obsessive-compulsive disorders.

4. Develop a plan of care from admission through discharge for a patient with an anxiety disorder. Be sure to include plans for education and follow-up.

CHAPTER

Mood Disorders

LEARNING OBJECTIVES

After studying this chapter, you should be able to:

♦ Discuss eight etiological theories of mood disorders.

♦ Identify six special treatment measures for mood disorders.

♦ Explain the primary behavioral characteristics of depressive and manic disorders.

♦ List the five primary NANDA nursing diagnoses appropriate for patients who experience mood disorders.

♦ Discuss nursing care outcomes and interventions for patients who experience mood disorders.

CHAPTER OVERVIEW

Mood disorders (depression and mania) are maladaptive responses to loss. Eight theories about their causes have been proposed. Nursing care for a patient with mood disorders focuses on preventing self-harm and meeting the patient's physical, behavioral, cognitive, emotional, and spiritual needs.

♦ **I. Introduction**

A. Description

1. A mood disorder is a severe disturbance in AFFECT manifested by extreme sadness or euphoria

2. Degrees of severity and duration vary

3. Maladaptive behavior may develop after a personal loss

4. Depression is commonly seen along with other psychiatric illnesses and with many major medical illnesses.

5. Heredity and environment play a role in development of mood disorders.

B. Classification

1. Etiology

   a. Exogenous: the result of external loss or event

   b. Endogenous: without apparent external cause

2. Symptomatology

   a. Reactive: a reaction to bereavement

   b. Endogenous: without apparent external cause

3. Activity

   a. Retarded

   b. Agitated

4. Mood changes

   a. Unipolar: only episodes of DEPRESSION

   b. Bipolar: MANIA alternating with depression

5. *DSM-IV* medical diagnoses

   a. Bipolar disorders, including manic and depressive disorders and cyclothymia

   b. Depressive disorders, including major depression and dysthymia

C. Etiology

1. Genetic

   a. Heritability is higher for bipolar disorders

   b. Mode of genetic transmission remains controversial

   c. Studies using genetic markers suggest that bipolar disorder is transmitted by the X-linked dominant gene

   d. Incidence is greater in relatives than in the general population

   e. The concordance rate is greater in monozygotic than in dizygotic twins

   f. Onset may occur without a precipitating stressor

2. Biological

   a. Neurotransmitter hypothesis

      (1) Catecholamine hypothesis

         (a) Biochemical studies show conflicting results regarding this hypothesis

         (b) Depression is caused by catecholamine deficiency

    (c) Mania is caused by catecholamine excess

    (d) Lag time between administration and effects of antide-
pressant medications does not support this hypothesis

  (2) Serotonin hypothesis

    (a) Concentrations of serotonin are low in mood disorders

    (b) Low concentrations of serotonin are found in people who
commit suicide

  (3) Dysregulation hypothesis

    (a) There is a generalized dysfunction in the mechanisms
that regulate neurotransmission at the synapses

    (b) Neurotransmitter systems interact with each other

    (c) Depression is associated with decreased activity within no-
repinephrine-serotonin component

    (d) Mania is associated with increased activity of no-
repinephrine-dopamine component

  (4) Gamma-aminobutyric acid (GABA) hypothesis

    (a) GABA modulates other neurotransmitter systems

    (b) Increased GABA activity has both an antidepressant and
an antimanic effect

  b. Endocrine dysfunction

    (1) Hypothalamic-pituitary-adrenal (HPA) axis

    (a) Stress activates HPA axis, which leads to secretion of corti-
sol

    (b) Many depressed patients secrete abnormally large
amounts of cortisol

    (c) Elevated levels of cortisol are not found in mania

    (2) Hypothalamic-pituitary-thyroid axis

    (a) Mood changes are often seen in thyroid disorders

    (b) Manic patients show blunted thyroid-stimulating hor-
mone response

    (3) Seasonality and circadian rhythms

    (a) Studies have linked seasonal variations in available sun-
light to changes in mood

    (b) Sleep cycle is linked to circadian rhythms of depressed
people

    (c) Rapid eye movement sleep of depressed people begins ear-
lier in the night and lasts twice as long as in nonde-
pressed individuals

    (d) Unclear whether changes in circadian rhythm cause or
are a result of changes in mood

3. Aggression-turned-inward theory (Sigmund Freud)

  a. Aggression accompanied by feelings of guilt

  b. Inability to express anger outwardly

  c. Validation of emotions unavailable empirically

4. Object-loss theory (J. Bowlby, R. Spitz, J. Robertson)
   a. Traumatic separation from significant persons or objects early in life
   b. Connection between early loss and adult depression unproven
5. Cognitive model (Aaron Beck)
   a. Depression resulting from negative view of self
   b. Negative evaluation of self, world, and future
   c. View of adverse event as a personal shortcoming; expectations of failure
   d. Dominated by pessimism
   e. Depression developing over weeks
   f. Model supported by clinical and experimental studies
6. Learned helplessness (Martin Seligman)
   a. Belief that no one will help and that one has no control over what happens
   b. Definition applies to a behavioral state and a personality trait
   c. Negative expectations lead to hopelessness, passivity, and nonassertiveness
   d. Syndrome cannot be empirically validated
7. Behavioral model (P. Lewinsohn)
   a. Depression caused by person-behavior-environment interaction
   b. Low rate of positive reinforcement or lack of rewarding interactions preceding depression
8. Stress factors
   a. Mood disturbances are a specific response to the stress of major life events or to accumulated minor stresses of daily living
   b. Stressors that may produce mood disturbances include:
      (1) Significant losses, such as death of a pet
      (2) Major life events, loss of self-esteem, interpersonal discord, socially undesirable occurrences, and major disruptions of life patterns
      (3) Role strain, such as single parent, student, caregiver
      (4) Physiologic changes in body function brought on by illness
   c. Stress theory is supported by research findings

D. Epidemiology
   1. Mood disorders are the most common psychiatric disorder
   2. Study of mood disorders is impeded by problems of definition and diagnosis
   3. Mood disorders are responsible for 75% of psychiatric hospitalizations and are prevalent in primary care situations
   4. Major depression is twice as common among women as among men
   5. Onset of unipolar disorder occurs in the mid- to late-thirties; bipolar disorders, in the late twenties
   6. Most untreated episodes of major depression last 6 to 24 months
   7. Most mood disorders increase risk of suicide

E. Special treatment measures
 1. Electroconvulsive therapy (ECT)
    a. This therapy requires a complete medical evaluation
    b. The patient must not eat or drink after midnight before therapy
    c. A nurse must remove the patient's shoes or slippers and any dentures or metal objects
    d. Anticholinergic medications are administered 30 minutes before the treatment begins
    e. An anesthesiologist administers oxygen, a short-acting anesthetic, and a muscle relaxant, and inserts an artificial airway before giving an electric charge
    f. The patient's arms should be restrained at the side
    g. Unilateral or bilateral electrodes are placed on the patient's frontal temporal regions
    h. The electric current produces a tonic seizure lasting 5 to 15 seconds and a clonic seizure lasting 10 to 60 seconds
    i. A usual course of therapy entails three treatments a week on alternate days
    j. The patient will experience confusion and forgetfulness, which usually disappear with time
    k. After treatment, the nurse should reorient the patient and record vital signs every 15 minutes until the patient is alert
 2. Psychopharmacologic treatment
    a. Antidepressant medication
       (1) No single medication is effective for all forms of depression
       (2) On the whole, therapeutic effects begin in 4 to 6 weeks after medication has begun
       (3) After remission, drugs are continued for 6 to 12 months to prevent a relapse
       (4) Categories of antidepressant drugs
           (a) Tricyclic drugs
           (b) Nontricyclic drugs
           (c) Selective serotonin reuptake inhibitors
           (d) Nonselective serotonin reuptake inhibitors
           (e) Monoamine oxidase inhibitors
    b. Antimanic medications
       (1) Lithium is useful in decreasing severity and frequency of depressive episodes
       (2) Lithium carbonate is used more frequently in children and adolescents
       (3) Examples include:
           (a) Carbamazepine (Tegretol)
           (b) Lithium carbonate (Eskalith)

(c) Lithium citrate (Cibalith-S)
(d) Valproic acid (Depakote)
3. Sleep manipulation
   a. Exact action is unknown
   b. Research shows that one night of sleep deprivation improves symptoms of depression
4. Phototherapy
   a. Treatment appears to be effective with *seasonal affective disorder*
   b. Treatment includes daily exposure to bright, artificial light for specified amount of time
   c. Improvement of symptoms is seen in 2 to 4 days
5. Group and individual therapies
   a. These therapies are less effective when used alone for major depression
   b. These therapies are more effective when combined with psychopharmacological treatment

♦ II. Diagnoses

A. Related *DSM-IV* medical diagnoses
1. Bipolar I disorder
2. Bipolar II disorder
3. Cyclothymic disorder
4. Major depressive disorder
5. Dysthymic disorder

B. Primary NANDA nursing diagnoses
1. Dysfunctional grieving
2. Hopelessness
3. Powerlessness
4. Spiritual distress
5. Risk for violence: self-directed

♦ III. Depressive reactions

A. Characteristics
1. Reactions range from mild and moderate to severe (major) states with or without psychotic features
2. Behaviors vary with level of severity
3. Change in usual behavior patterns is key aspect of assessment
4. Most common behavior reported is depressed mood
5. Anxiety is often seen in depressed individuals
6. Subgroups of major depressive disorders include
   a. Psychotic
   b. Melancholic
   c. Atypical

     d. Seasonal

     e. Postpartum psychosis

     f. Postpartum depression

B. Nursing assessment

  1. Complete in short time segments because thinking is slowed in depressed individuals; important to determine the severity of the patient's depression (See *Determining the severity of a patient's depression,* page 74)

  2. Collect data including

     a. Affective, behavioral, cognitive and physiologic manifestations (See *Manifestations of depression,* page 75)

     b. Precipitating stressors

     c. Past psychiatric history

     d. Medical history

     e. Mental status

     f. Suicidal ideation

     g. Coping mechanisms

     h. Support systems

C. Nursing planning and implementation

  1. Outcomes

     a. Patient will maintain an adequate balance of nutrition, hydration, elimination, rest, sleep, and activity

     b. Patient will not harm self or others

     c. Patient will express feelings of self-worth

     d. Patient will acquire adaptive coping responses to stressors

  2. Nursing interventions: Physical needs

     a. Monitor and record nutritional intake

     b. Weigh the patient daily

     c. Encourage small, frequent high-fiber meals and foods easily chewed; stay with patient during meals

     d. Teach methods to help the patient relax and sleep

     e. Assist patient in getting out of bed and taking care of personal hygiene; encourage the patient to initiate self-care

     f. Encourage exercise to prevent constipation; administer laxatives as needed

     g. Provide opportunities for exercise

CLINICAL ALERT

     h. Give help in a matter-of-fact manner

     i. Assess the risk of suicide; the potential for self directed violence is high for any patient with depression but the risk increases with the severity of the depression

     j. Observe the patient for medication compliance and side effects

DECISION TREE
Determining the severity of a patient's depression

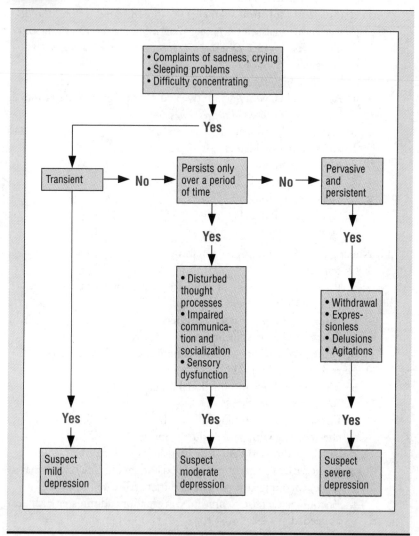

3. Nursing interventions: Behavioral needs
   a. Mobilize the patient to productive activity by assigning therapeutic tasks
   b. Provide opportunities for increased involvement in activities through a structured, daily program
   c. Select activities that ensure success and accomplishment
   d. Help the patient enhance social skills

Manifestations of depression

Use the chart below to help distinguish the different manifestations for each level of depression.

	Affective manifestations	Cognitive manifestations	Physiologic manifestations	Behavioral manifestations
Mild depression	• Sadness	• Decreased alertness • Difficulty thinking logically and concentrating	• Altered sleep patterns	• Crying • Irritability • Increased use of alcohol or drugs
Moderate depression	• Despondency • Dejection • Gloom • Low self-esteem • Powerlessness • Helplessness • Inability to experience pleasure (potential for suicide attempt)	• Slowed thinking • Narrowing of interests and indecisiveness • Self-doubt • Rumination • Pessimism	• Somatic complaints • Anorexia • Weight loss • Fatigue • Sleep disturbance	• Withdrawal • Tears • Irritability • Poor hygiene • Slow movement and speech • Agitation • Increased use of alcohol or drugs
Severe depression	• Despair • Hopelessness • Worthlessness • Guilt • Valuelessness • Loneliness	• Confusion and indecisiveness • Inability to concentrate • Lack of motivation • Intense self-blame and deprecation • Wish to die • Possible delusions or hallucinations	• Constipation • Urine retention • Amenorrhea • Lack of sexual interest • Impotence • Marked weight loss • Insomnia	• Psychomotor retardation • Poor posture • Decreased speech • Slow responses • Unkempt appearance • Social withdrawal

4. Nursing interventions: Cognitive needs
   a. Increase self-esteem and sense of control over behavior
   b. Modify negative expectations and explore the extent of negative thinking
   c. Help patient substitute positive thoughts for negative ones
   d. Educate patient and family about mood disorders (See *Patient with depression,* page 76)
   e. Establish realistic goals

TEACHING TIPS
Patient with depression

Be sure to include the following topics in your teaching plan for the patient with depression.
- Definition of depression
- Symptoms of depression
- Impact of symptoms on social interactions and relationships
- Antidepressant medication: benefits, usage, dosage, and side effects
- Coping with depression
- Early signs of relapse and role of compliance
- Coping with stress
- Dealing with suicide threat and attempt
- Use of community resources

5. Nursing interventions: Emotional needs
  a. Slowly and cautiously make the patient aware of unconscious feelings
  b. Plan activities that allow for physical sublimation of aggressive feelings
  c. Talk about the universality of feelings
  d. Encourage constructive expression when the patient discusses anger
  e. Provide hope
  f. Assess yourself: depression can be contagious
6. Nursing interventions: Spiritual needs
  a. Assess the patient's loss of belief
  b. Help the patient explore spiritual beliefs or a meaningful philosophy of life
  c. Arrange for a spiritual advisor to visit, if appropriate
D. Evaluation
  1. Use observation and the patient's reports as a basis for evaluation
  2. Note goal accomplishments
  3. Note patient growth in insight and development of alternate coping skills
  4. Keep in mind the depressed patient's reluctance to acknowledge progress
  5. Complete a nursing self-assessment

♦ **IV. Manic reactions**

A. Nursing assessment
  1. Characteristics
    a. The condition usually develops more rapidly than depressive reactions
    b. Patient fails to view behavior as inappropriate

  c. The maladaptive behavior is a defense against depression
 2. Physical manifestations
  a. Deteriorated physical appearance
  b. Increased energy; feeling of being "charged up"
  c. Increased sexual interest and activity
  d. Decreased sleep disturbance
 3. Emotional manifestations
  a. Mood lability; euphoria
  b. Feelings of grandiosity
  c. Inflated sense of self-worth
 4. Cognitive manifestations
  a. Difficulty concentrating
  b. Flight of ideas
  c. Delusions of grandeur
  d. Impaired judgment
 5. Behavioral manifestations
  a. Rapid, jumbled speech
  b. Hyperactivity
  c. Impulsiveness, lack of inhibition, recklessness
  d. Increased social contacts
  e. Hypersexuality
  f. Verbosity; often rhyming and punning
  g. Bizarre and eccentric appearance
B. Nursing planning and implementation
 1. Outcomes
  a. Patient will not harm self or others
  b. Patient will maintain an adequate balance of rest, sleep, and nutrition
  c. Patient will comply with treatment
  d. Patient will monitor own behavior and exercise self-control
 2. Nursing interventions: Physical needs
  a. Decrease environmental stimuli by acting as a consistent caregiver who supplies external controls
  b. Offer finger foods
  c. Encourage short rest periods
  d. Enforce minimal standards of personal hygiene
  e. Monitor medications
  f. Monitor elimination
 3. Nursing interventions: Behavioral needs
  a. Suggest sedentary activities, and offer motor activities in moderation
  b. Define and explain acceptable behaviors, then set limits
  c. Negotiate limits on demanding, manipulative behaviors
  d. Avoid frustrating the patient unnecessarily
  e. Safeguard the patient from physical risks

4. Nursing interventions: Cognitive needs
   a. Discourage the patient from expensive purchases
   b. Help the patient identify behaviors that lead to a manic episode
   c. Explore effects of behavior on others
   d. Intervene when the patient has *delusions*
   e. Increase the patient's self-esteem
5. Nursing interventions: Emotional needs
   a. Help the patient become aware of underlying anger
   b. Help patient verbally acknowledge resistance to therapy
   c. Teach the patient to make decisions and accept responsibility
6. Nursing interventions: Spiritual needs
   a. Help the patient explore a meaningful philosophy of life
   b. Arrange for a spiritual advisor to visit, if appropriate

C. Evaluation
   1. Use observation and the patient's reports as a basis for evaluation
   2. Note goal accomplishment
   3. Note patient growth in insight and development of alternate coping skills
   4. Complete a nursing self-assessment

POINTS TO REMEMBER

◆ Alterations in mood are common responses to life changes.

◆ Mood disorders are maladaptive responses to loss characterized by extreme disturbances in affect.

◆ No single etiology of mood disorders has been universally accepted or empirically validated.

◆ All patients with mood disorders should be assessed for suicide risk.

◆ Nursing care outcomes and interventions vary, depending on the patient and the disorder, and should be carefully adapted to the individual following assessment.

STUDY QUESTIONS

To evaluate your understanding of this chapter, answer the following questions in the space provided; then compare your responses with the correct answers in Appendix B, pages 170 and 171.

1. What are the five biologic etiologies for mood disorders? _____

   _____

   _____

2. Who developed the learned helplessness concept as an etiology for mood
   disorders?_____

   _____

   _____

3. What are the six special treatment measures for mood disorders? _____

   _____

   _____

4. Which cognitive changes will the nurse observe when a patient is experiencing moderate depression? _____

   _____

   _____

5. When a patient is experiencing depression, which nursing intervention is
   most important in meeting the patient's physical needs? _____

   _____

   _____

6. What are the primary nursing outcomes when caring for a manic patient?

   _____

   _____

CRITICAL THINKING AND APPLICATION EXERCISES

1. Develop a table comparing the biological theories of mood disorders.

2. Observe an ECT. Prepare an oral presentation describing the treatment.
   Also describe nursing care before, during, and after treatment.

3. Prepare cards describing lithium, valproic acid, and carbamazepine.

4. Research monoamine oxidase inhibitors. Develop a patient instruction
   sheet for this class of drugs.

5. Develop a plan of care from admission through discharge for a patient
   with a mood disorder. Be sure to include plans for education and follow-up.

CHAPTER

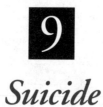

Suicide

LEARNING OBJECTIVES

After studying this chapter, you should be able to:

♦ Describe eight common myths of suicide.

♦ Identify groups at high risk for suicidal behavior.

♦ Describe the physical, emotional, cognitive, and behavioral characteristics of a suicidal individual.

♦ Complete a nursing assessment of a suicidal patient.

♦ Formulate a nursing care plan for a hospitalized suicidal patient.

CHAPTER OVERVIEW

Five theories have been proposed to explain SUICIDE— the ultimate form of SELF-DESTRUCTIVE BEHAVIOR. Certain factors have been identified as placing a patient at high risk for suicide. Nursing care of the suicidal patient focuses on protecting the patient from self-harm, helping the patient develop adaptive coping mechanisms, and ensuring compliance with treatment.

♦ I. Introduction

A. Description
   1. The ultimate form of self-destructive behavior, suicide is condemned in most societies and illegal in some states
   2. Depending on its severity, SUICIDAL IDEATION can take the form of a threat, a gesture, or an attempt
   3. Suicidal intent is commonly signaled by mood swings, decline in job performance, and withdrawal from family and friends
   4. Suicide is not necessarily the act of someone who is mentally ill

B. Epidemiology
   1. Statistics reflect incomplete reporting
   2. More women than men attempt suicide
   3. More men than women are successful at committing suicide
   4. Suicide accounts for 1% of all deaths each year
   5. It is the 10th leading cause of death for all ages and the 3rd leading cause of death between the ages of 15 to 24
   6. The highest suicide rate in the U.S. is among people over 65.
   7. Incidence of suicide is higher in urban areas
   8. Suicide tends to be seasonal, with the highest number occurring in April and May and the lowest in December
   9. Suicide occurs most frequently on Fridays, Sundays, and Mondays
   10. It is 500 times more prevalent among people with serious depressive reactions
   11. Suicide is more common among caucasians
   12. 90% of adults who commit suicide have an associated psychiatric illness

C. Myths about suicide
   1. People who talk about suicide don't do it
   2. Suicide happens without warning
   3. Suicidal people wish to die
   4. Once someone becomes suicidal, the person is always suicidal
   5. Once a person's depression has lifted, the danger of suicide is over
   6. Suicide is inherited and runs in families
   7. Suicidal people are mentally ill
   8. If someone is despondent, mentioning suicide will give the person suicidal ideas

D. Theories of suicidal behavior
   1. Psychodynamic
      a. Hostile feelings turned inward
      b. Loss of self-esteem resulting from self-condemnation and guilt
      c. Ego withdrawal resulting from stress
      d. Attempt to gain immortality, maintain ego, or solve an identification conflict

Neurobiological
1. Suicidal behaviors are linked to decreased serotonin levels
2. Suicidal behaviors are associated with decreased dopaminergic neurotransmission
3. Socioeconomic
   a. Painful or life-threatening illness
   b. Inadequate integration into society
   c. Relationship between psychodynamic, cultural, ethnic, and social factors
4. Communication
   a. Form of communication or aggressive retaliation
   b. Way of relieving guilt
5. Sociopsychological
   a. Result of unsatisfactory relationships or breakup of satisfactory relationships
   b. Outcome of unsatisfactory social interaction
   c. Effort to solve problems of living
   d. Response to crisis
   e. Peak times for suicide during adolescence and old age

◆ II. Nursing assessment: High-risk groups

A. Risk factors
   1. Previous attempts
      a. Best predictor of suicide
      b. Need to be asked about directly
   2. Depression
      a. 3 to 12 times greater risk
      b. Predictor is hopelessness
   3. Schizophrenia
      a. Risk is increased with command hallucinations
      b. 15% commit suicide
   4. LETHALITY
      a. Risk increases if plan is well-developed
      b. Risk increases if planned means is available
      c. Risk depends on level of intent
   5. Substance abuse
      a. Impairs judgment
      b. Increases impulsivity
   6. Major health problems
      a. Terminal illness
      b. Chronic illness
      c. Rejection of or noncompliance with treatment

7. Age
   a. Third leading cause of death in children and adolescents
   b. Older adults have higher rates of successful suicides
8. Gender
   a. More women attempt suicide
   b. More males actually kill themselves
9. Personality traits
   a. Hostile, impulsive, or aggressor
   b. Hopeless
   c. Low self-esteem
   d. Negative and rigid thinking
10. Psychosocial stressors
   a. Recent loss (such as divorce)
   b. Unemployed
   c. Socially isolated
   d. Multiple life stressors

B. Patient behaviors and dynamics
1. Physical manifestations
   a. Depression in about 75% of cases
   b. Vague, nonspecific somatic complaints
   c. Persistent insomnia
   d. Weight loss
   e. Slowed speech
2. Emotional manifestations
   a. Worthlessness
   b. Helplessness
   c. Hopelessness
   d. Ambivalence
   e. Anxiety
   f. Fear
   g. Excessive guilt
   h. Self-blame
   i. Frustration
   j. Anger
   k. Emotional calmness
3. Cognitive manifestations
   a. Preoccupation with self-harm
   b. Desire to escape untenable life situation
   c. DICHOTOMOUS THINKING
   d. SEMANTIC FALLACIES (for example, "Tom ignored me; that must mean I'm no good")
4. Behavioral manifestations
   a. Sudden behavioral changes
   b. Decision to put affairs in order

      c. Disclosure of coded or direct messages (for example, "I won't be seeing you again.")

◆ III. Diagnoses

A. Related *DSM-IV* medical diagnoses
1. Bipolar disorder
2. Borderline personality disorder
3. Major depressive disorder
4. Noncompliance with treatment
5. Schizophrenia
6. Substance use disorders

B. Primary NANDA diagnostic categories
1. Risk for self-mutilation
2. Noncompliance
3. Risk for violence: self-directed

◆ IV. Treatment modalities

A. Outpatient crisis intervention

B. Inpatient hospitalization

C. Pharmacologic agents
1. Antidepressant agents
2. Antianxiety agents
3. Antimanic agents

D. Electroconvulsive therapy (ECT)

◆ V. Nursing planning and implementation

A. General comments
1. Primary focus is on protecting person from self-harm
2. Need to address underlying reasons for suicidal behavior

B. Outcomes
1. Patient will not harm self
2. Patient will comply with treatment
3. Patient will develop adaptive coping mechanisms

C. Interventions for the hospitalized patient
1. Provide a safe environment, and protect the patient from self-harm
    a. Determine the appropriate level of suicide precautions, and explain them to the patient
    b. Assess the patient's suicide potential at least daily
    c. Evaluate the level of precautions daily
    d. Obtain assessment data in a matter-of-fact manner
    e. Ask the patient directly about the suicide plan

    f. Remove dangerous objects

    g. Place the patient in a room near the nurses' station in view of staff

    h. Make sure the windows are locked

    i. Stay with the patient when sharp objects must be used

2. Maintain close supervision

    a. Know the whereabouts of the patient at all times

    b. Stay with the patient during bathing, shaving, and similar activities

    c. Check the patient frequently at irregular intervals through the night

    d. Be especially alert when the staff is reduced (change of shift, holidays, weekends)

    e. Observe and note behavior patterns

    f. Be aware of manipulative or attention-seeking behavior

CLINICAL ALERT

3. Be alert to the possibility that the patient is either saving or not taking medications. Stay with the patient while the patient is taking medications, and check the mouth after swallowing to ensure that drug is not hidden under the tongue or in the buccal pouch

    a. Observe and report sudden changes in mood; a sudden calmness or lifting of depression may indicate that the patient has decided on suicide and formulated a plan

    b. Avoid promising not to tell

    c. Watch for decreased communication, conversations about death, disorientation, dependency, or concealing of articles

4. Place limits on RUMINATION about suicide; discuss the patient's emotions but not the previous attempts

5. Prevent the patient from harming others

6. Promote adequate nutrition, hydration, and elimination

7. Promote a balance of rest, sleep, and activity

8. Reduce feelings of depression; encourage feelings of self-worth

    a. Convey caring

    b. Encourage the patient to express feelings

    c. Do not joke about death

    d. Do not belittle previous attempts

    e. Provide opportunities for successful accomplishment of tasks or goals to enhance the patient's self-worth

    f. Help the patient identify positive aspects of the self

    g. Involve the patient, if possible, in planning treatment

9. Reduce withdrawal from people

    a. Seek out the patient for conversation

    b. Encourage the patient to spend time away from the hospital room

    c. Promote group interaction as appropriate

10. Help the patient develop insight into his relationships with others

TEACHING TIPS
Family of a suicidal patient

Be sure to include the following topics in your teaching plan for the family of a patient who is suicidal.
- Possible risk factors for suicide
- Role of stress in suicide
- Signs and symptoms of depression
- Manifestations of possible suicidal behavior
- Myths about suicide
- Need for follow up
- Supportive services

11. Increase the patient's ability to deal with future suicidal feelings; instruct patient and family about suicide (See *Family of a suicidal patient*)
    a. Review hypothetical situations
    b. Plan how to recognize and deal with feelings and situations that have caused stress
12. Complete a nursing self-assessment (include thoughts and feelings evoked by patient and ability to be an effective care giver)

D. Interventions for families following a suicide
    1. Lessen long-term effects and promote grieving
    2. Recognize that support from friends is commonly lacking
    3. Help the family explore their guilt
    4. Be alert to an "anniversary suicide" by a survivor
    5. Help the family deal with hostility and destructiveness

♦ **VI. Evaluation**

A. PSYCHOLOGICAL AUTOPSY (review of the patient's life to determine whether anything could have been done to prevent suicide)

B. Nursing self-assessment regarding feelings and thoughts about suicide, the person who committed suicide, and about effectiveness of interventions as a care giver

POINTS TO REMEMBER

♦ Suicide is more prevalent among those with severe depressive reactions; suicide is not necessarily the act of someone who is mentally ill.

♦ Common characteristics of suicidal persons are ambivalence, guilt, helplessness, hopelessness, loneliness, and a lack of future orientation.

♦ The major nursing care outcome for a suicidal patient is to provide a safe environment and protect the patient from self-harm.

♦ The nurse must be prepared to ask direct questions about the patient's suicidal thoughts and plans.

STUDY QUESTIONS

To evaluate your understanding of this chapter, answer the following questions in the space provided; then compare your responses with the correct answers in Appendix B, page 171.

1. What are risk factors associated with suicidal behavior? _____

   _____

   _____

2. What are the three categories of pharmacologic agents used to treat suicidal patients? _____

   _____

   _____

3. Which interventions would a nurse use to create a safe environment and protect the patient from harm? _____

   _____

   _____

4. Which nursing interventions are important when caring for the families of after a suicide? _____

   _____

   _____

CRITICAL THINKING AND APPLICATION EXERCISES

1. Perform a self-assessment for suicide risk using the identified risk factors.

2. Review your health care institution's policy regarding suicide precautions.

3. With two or three classmates, role play about dealing with a friend's suicide.

4. Care for a patient with suicidal behavior. Develop a specific plan of care including education and follow-up.

CHAPTER

10

Schizophrenic Disorders

LEARNING OBJECTIVES

After studying this chapter, you should be able to:

♦ Define psychotic behavior.

♦ Describe four theories that explain the etiology of schizophrenia.

♦ Describe four manifestations of various types of schizophrenia.

♦ Identify nursing diagnoses appropriate to the schizophrenic patient.

♦ Develop a nursing care plan for the schizophrenic patient.

CHAPTER OVERVIEW

A difference in the perception of reality characterizes psychotic behavior. Schizophrenia refers to a group of disorders manifested by changes in cognitive, perceptual, affective, motor, and social domains. Nursing assessment focuses on identifying the primary, cognitive, linguistic, perceptual, affective, behavioral, and social manifestations seen in the schizophrenic patient. Nursing interventions focus on promoting patient safety, meeting the patient's physical needs, and helping the patient deal with reality. Specific interventions are necessary for dealing with delusions and hallucinations.

♦ I. Psychotic behavior

A. PSYCHOTIC BEHAVIOR includes various symptoms resulting from disturbed thought processes, distorted PERCEPTIONS, brain damage, chemical toxicity, or maladaptive neurobiological responses

B. The psychotic person perceives reality differently from most people and has difficulty evaluating reality

♦ II. Schizophrenia

A. General comments
  1. Schizophrenia refers to a brain illness of unknown etiology
  2. Schizophrenics experience a split between thought and affect and a split with reality
  3. Schizophrenia categorizes a group of disorders manifested by changes in the cognitive, perceptual, affective, motor, and social domains
  4. Schizophrenia is characterized by remissions and exacerbations

B. Causative theories
  1. Genetic factors
     a. Biological relatives of persons with schizophrenia are at greater risk
     b. About 40% to 50% of identical twins and 9% to 10% of fraternal twins are schizophrenic
     c. Vulnerability to schizophrenia increases with closeness of biological relationship
     d. Monogenic theory assumes transmission of a single gene that produces susceptibility to schizophrenia; under stress, the carrier is likely to become schizophrenic
     e. Polygenic theory assumes causation by inheritance of more than one gene
     f. Social or environmental stress may contribute to the onset of the disorder by interacting with the person's inherited biological makeup
  2. Neurobiological theories
     a. Brain abnormalities causing maladaptive neurobiological responses have recently been found
        (1) The third ventricle of prefrontal system is larger on the left side
        (2) Gray matter is decreased in the temporal lobe
        (3) Blood flow is decreased to the frontal lobes
        (4) Glucose metabolism is decreased in the temporal and frontal lobes
        (5) Lesions occur in the amygdala region
        (6) Glucose metabolism is increased in the basal ganglia

  b. Neurotransmitters are thought to be involved
    (1) Hyperactivity in dopamine system may produce systems such as delusions and hallucinations
    (2) Defect in selective neuropinephrene neuron degeneration may be related to ANHEDONIA, social withdrawal, and flat affect
    (3) Serotonin elevation may cause hallucinations
    (4) Diminished levels of gamma-aminobutyric acid (GABA) may inhibit dopamine activity
    (5) Higher fasting serum phenylketonurea levels have been found
3. Developmental theories
  a. The disorder starts early in life when the relationship between the child and the primary caregiver is impaired or inadequate
  b. Deficient nurturing results in difficulty learning to interact with others and an inability to trust oneself or others
  c. The theory focuses on the child's need to receive and give love
  d. The child is traumatized by a lack or an unpredictability of maternal love
  e. Symbiotic relationships prevent normal maturation
  f. Schizophrenogenic mothers have been described as overinvolved, yet anxious, ungiving, and unpredictable
  g. Schizophrenogenic fathers have been described as weak, ineffectual role models
  h. In schizophrenogenic families, relationships are intricate and confusing
4. Psychodynamic theories
  a. Schizophrenia may be preceded by the formation of a fragile ego, which cannot withstand the demands of external reality
  b. Conflicts arise when a disparity exists between psychological needs and sociocultural expectations
  c. The relationship with the mother is marked by ambivalence
  d. Difficulty separating from the mother may be a factor in the disorder's onset

C. Sequential steps of the schizophrenic process
  1. Inability to trust
  2. Dissociation
  3. Displacement
  4. Fantasy
  5. Projection

D. Types and subtypes
  1. Catatonic type
    a. Least common
    b. Little reaction to environment
    c. Excitement at times
    d. Bizarre postures

      2. Disorganized type
        a. Silly affect
        b. Incoherent thought
        c. Loose associations
        d. Disorganized behavior
      3. Paranoid type
        a. Systematized delusions
        b. Auditory hallucinations
        c. Easily angered
        d. High risk for violence
      4. Residual type
        a. Emotional blunting
        b. Eccentric behavior
        c. Loose association
        d. Social withdrawal
      5. Undifferentiated type
        a. Delusions
        b. Hallucinations
        c. Disorganized behavior

♦ III. Treatment modalities

A. Psychopharmacology
    1. Antipsychotic medications
    2. Antiparkinsonian medications (for side effects of neuroleptics)

B. RELATIONSHIP THERAPY

C. Group therapy

D. Individual psychotherapy

E. MILIEU THERAPY

F. Family therapy

G. Supportive psychotherapy

H. Psychoeducational programs (See *Patient with schizophrenia and his family,* page 92)

I. Social skills training

J. Stress management

♦ IV. Nursing assessment

A. Primary manifestations
    1. Associative looseness
        a. Inability to organize thoughts logically
        b. Inability to pursue a single concept to a logical conclusion

TEACHING TIPS
Patient with schizophrenia and his family

Be sure to include the following topics in your teaching plan for the patient with schizophrenia and his family:
- Definition of schizophrenia and psychosis
- Myths about schizophrenia
- Schizophrenia as a medical illness
- Symptoms and usual course of schizophrenia
- Antipsychotic medications: benefits, usage, dosages, and side effects
- Relationship between anxiety and stress and psychosis
- Coping with stress
- Early signs of relapse
- Role of compliance
- Listening and communicating skills
- Dealing with hallucinations, illusions, noncompliance, use of alcohol or drugs
- Use of community resources

    c. Unrelated thoughts
    d. Irrelevant ideas
    e. MAGICAL THINKING
  2. AUTISTIC THINKING
    a. Form of subjective thinking
    b. Reliance on a personal and illogical interpretation of reality
    c. Thinking not validated by objective reality
    d. Fantasy and daydreaming as substitutes for reality
    e. Minimal distinction between the self and the environment
    f. Personal meanings applied to persons and events
  3. Ambivalence
    a. Conflicting feelings toward self, significant others, situations, events, and relationships
    b. Negativism; repetitive, ceaseless, nonmeaningful activity; over-compliance; apathy; or immobilization
  4. Alterations of affect
    a. Protective actions
    b. Inappropriate affect: outward display is not in harmony with real-ity
    c. Blunted affect: extreme decrease in the intensity of response
    d. Apathy: indifference to the environment characterized by a lack of commitment and involvement
B. Cognitive manifestations
  1. Concrete thinking
  2. Blocked speech

3. Poverty of speech and ideas

4. Symbolic associations

5. TANGENTIALITY

6. STEREOTYPED SPEECH

7. DELUSIONS

   a. May include grandeur, persecution, reference, influence, and somatic types

   b. Develop through stages of anxiety, denial, projection, and rationalization

   c. Reflect an underlying need to deny unacceptable feelings about the self

C. Linguistic manifestations

1. ECHOLALIA

2. CLANG ASSOCIATION

3. NEOLOGISM

4. WORD SALAD

5. MUTISM

D. Perceptual manifestations: HALLUCINATIONS

1. Are false sensory perceptions with no basis in reality, generated by internal rather than external stimuli

2. Include auditory, gustatory, olfactory, tactile, visual, and somatic hallucinations

3. Develop in three phases

   a. The patient focuses on comforting thoughts to relieve anxiety and stress

   b. The patient projects these comforting thoughts to external objects

   c. The patient experiences increasing preoccupation and helplessness; the hallucination is controlling but comforting, although content may become menacing

4. May become chronic if no intervention occurs

E. Affective manifestations

1. Overresponse

2. Blunted AFFECT

3. Lack of affect

4. Lability

F. Alterations in body image

1. Depersonalization

   a. Lack of ego boundaries

   b. Feelings of unreality and instability about the self

   c. Sense of living in a dream

   d. Inability to discriminate between the inner and outer parts of one's body

      e. Loss of self-control

      f. Sense of merging with the environment

  2. Identity confusion

      a. Loss of orientation in space

      b. Inability to recognize sexual identity

  3. Hypochondriasis

      a. Intense self-focus

      b. Preoccupation with bodily sensations and functions

      c. Physical symptoms with no basis in reality

G. Behavioral manifestations

  1. Withdrawal

  2. Regression

  3. Overactivity or underactivity

  4. Impulsivity

  5. Ritualistic mannerisms

  6. AUTOMATION

  7. Stereotypy (rigid categorization or structure)

H. Social manifestations

  1. Anxiety associated with relatedness (inability to establish intimate relationships) plus autistic thinking

  2. Loneliness

      a. Estrangement

      b. Emptiness, barrenness, and despair

  3. Social isolation

      a. Intense shyness to complete reclusiveness

      b. Dependent on the degree of anxiety generated by interaction

  4. Superficial relationships

      a. Mistrust of others

      b. Perception of others as unauthentic, unreliable, and dangerous

  5. Dependence

      a. Excessive reliance on others

      b. Manipulation of others by repeated demands

◆ V. Related diagnoses

A. Related *DSM-IV* medical diagnoses

  1. Schizophrenic

      a. Paranoid type

      b. Disorganized type

      c. Catatonic type

      d. Undifferentiated type

      e. Residual type

  2. Schizophreniform disorder

  3. Schizoaffective disorder

4. Delusional disorder
5. Brief psychotic disorder
6. Shared psychotic disorder

B. Related primary NANDA nursing diagnoses
1. Impaired verbal communication
2. Sensory or perceptual alteration
3. Impaired social interaction
4. Social isolation
5. Altered thought processes

♦ **VI. Nursing planning and implementation**

A. Problem and need identification
1. Priority problems commonly relate to basic physical and safety needs in an acute psychotic episode
2. Problems are interrelated; the etiology of one problem may, in itself, be a separate problem
3. Not all symptoms are separate problems
4. Problems should be grouped in related concepts

B. Principles of nursing care
1. Unless educationally prepared to conduct group or family therapy, the nurse generalist uses RELATIONSHIP THERAPY
2. Nurse must convey a sincere wish to understand and communicate
3. Principles of therapeutic interaction include:
a. Acceptance of patient
b. Acknowledgment
c. Authenticity
d. Self-awareness
4. Trust is essential to effective nursing care

C. Outcomes
1. Patient will demonstrate increased level of functioning
2. Patient will demonstrate increased sense of well-being
3. Patient will successfully manage symptoms

D. General nursing interventions
1. Provide a safe environment
a. Briefly explain procedures, routines, and tests
b. Protect the patient from self-destructive tendencies
2. Monitor physical needs; maintain adequate nutrition, hydration, and elimination
3. Decrease withdrawn behavior
a. Spend time with the patient
b. Do not make unrealistic promises
c. Teach the patient that feelings are valid

      d. Limit the patient's environment

      e. Maintain staff consistency

      f. Begin with one-on-one interactions, then progress to small groups

      g. Establish a daily routine

  4. Increase the patient's self-esteem

      a. Provide attention in a sincere manner

      b. Offer praise

      c. Avoid trying to convince the patient of worth verbally

      d. Assist the patient with activities of daily living

  5. Orient the patient to reality

  6. Help the patient establish ego boundaries

      a. Validate the patient's real perceptions

      b. Correct misconceptions in a matter-of-fact manner

      c. Do not argue

      d. Stay with the frightened patient

      e. Discuss simple, concrete topics

      f. Provide activities that maintain contact with reality

  7. Maintain a safe, therapeutic environment for other patients

      a. Remove the patient from the group when necessary

      b. Help the group accept the patient's behavior

      c. Make sure that at least one staff member attends to other patients

      d. Explain to other patients that the patient's behavior is a result of illness and not of anything they did

  8. Help the patient work through regressive behavior

      a. Assess the present level of functioning, and communicate with the patient at that level

      b. Encourage more adult behavior

      c. Help identify unmet needs or feelings

      d. Encourage the expression of feelings

      e. Set realistic goals and expectations daily

      f. Make the patient aware of expectations

      g. Initially, make choices for the patient

      h. Gradually, offer the patient opportunities to make decisions and accept responsibility

  9. Reduce bizarre behavior, anxiety, agitation, or aggression

      a. Set limits on behavior

      b. Reduce excessive stimuli

      c. Give medication as needed

E. Interventions for delusions

  1. Provide sensitivity

CLINICAL
ALERT
∎

  2. Avoid supporting or reinforcing the delusion

  3. Do not directly attack the delusion; this will increase anxiety

  4. Express doubt tactfully

  5. Recognize delusion as the patient's perception of the environment

6. Focus on reality
7. Avoid judging
8. Empathize with the patient's feelings and help the person deal with underlying needs or feelings in a healthy way
9. Maintain homeostasis

F. Interventions for hallucinations
   1. Assess the underlying unmet need
   2. Establish trust
   3. Recognize and acknowledge the affective component
   4. Be alert for clues that the patient is hallucinating
   5. Cast doubt tactfully
   6. Discuss reality-based issues
   7. Protect the patient from self-harm or harm to others or objects
   8. Reduce stimuli
   9. Communicate in direct, concrete, specific terms
   10. Provide simple activities
   11. Evaluate the patient's ability to tolerate touch
   12. Provide a structured environment
   13. Assess signs of increasing fear, anxiety, or agitation
   14. Intervene appropriately (for example, with one-on-one contact, seclusion, medication)
   15. Do not corner the patient
   16. Help the patient express feelings
   17. Help the patient deal with guilt, remorse, or embarrassment when he remembers psychotic behavior
   18. Help the patient deal with possible recurrence of hallucinations

♦ **VII. Evaluation**

A. Document progress for the patient
B. Be realistic; expect change to be slow
C. Modify the care plan as needed

POINTS TO REMEMBER

♦ Statistics on the incidence and prevalence of schizophrenia are unreliable because of disagreements about diagnosis. Etiologic explanations of schizophrenia remain inconclusive but current research is focusing on neurobiological explanations.

♦ Primary symptoms of altered patterns of thought and perception include ambivalence, autism, altered affect, and loose associations.

♦ The use of antipsychotic medication has enabled many schizophrenics to participate in other therapies and to function outside the hospital.

♦ Nurses must help patients and families understand the need for medication.

♦ Relationship therapy is the most suitable therapy for generalist nurses working with schizophrenic patients.

STUDY QUESTIONS

To evaluate your understanding of this chapter, answer the following questions in the space provided; then compare your responses with the correct answers in Appendix B, pages 171 and 172.

1. What is psychotic behavior? _____

_____

_____

2. What are the sequential steps of the schizophrenic process? _____

_____

_____

3. Which primary manifestations are identified during assessment of a patient with schizophrenia? _____

_____

_____

4. How do perceptual manifestations (hallucinations) develop? _____

_____

_____

5. What are four behavioral manifestations that the nurse might see when assessing the patient with schizophrenia? _____

_____

_____

6. What is the priority problem in an acute psychotic episode? _____

_____

_____

7. What are the principles of therapeutic interaction? _____

_____

_____

8. How would a nurse help a patient establish ego boundaries? _____

_____

_____

CRITICAL THINKING AND APPLICATION EXERCISES

1. Develop a table listing the different types of hallucinations; provide realistic examples for each.

2. Compare and contrast the causative theories about schizophrenia.

3. Research antipsychotic agents; prepare drug cards for the major ones.

4. Develop a plan of care for a patient with schizophrenia; include education and follow-up.

Personality Disorders: Maladaptive Social Responses

LEARNING OBJECTIVES

After studying this chapter, you should be able to:

♦ Identify at least six characteristics of a healthy interpersonal relationship.

♦ Discuss predisposing factors that contribute to maladaptive social responses.

♦ Formulate individual nursing diagnoses for patients with personality disorders.

♦ Identify nursing interventions for patients with personality disorders.

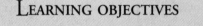

CHAPTER OVERVIEW

Personality disorders are viewed in relation to maladaptive social responses that result in disrupted social relatedness. Certain characteristics can be identified as risk factors for developing personality disorders. Nursing interventions focus on dealing with the manifested behaviors rather than reacting to them.

◆ I. Adaptive social responses

A. Characteristics of healthy interpersonal relationships
1. Intimacy while maintaining separate identities
2. Sensitivity to needs of another
3. Mutual validation of personal worth
4. Open communication of feelings
5. Acceptance of another as a valued, separate person
6. Deep EMPATHY
7. Willingness to risk self-revelation
8. Ability and willingness to subordinate one's needs to those of another or to the demands of a relationship
9. Interdependency
10. EGO-SYNTONIC BEHAVIOR

B. Development of relatedness throughout the life cycle
1. Infancy
   a. The infant depends on others
   b. The infant's trust develops as a result of a consistent, reliable relationship with a significant other
2. Childhood
   a. The child strives to establish the self as a separate individual
   b. Parental love and consistent limit-setting communicate caring
   c. The child develops a capacity for interdependence
   d. Parental guidelines for behavior are internalized
   e. A value system emerges
   f. Peer relationships and approval of adults outside the family group become important
3. Preadolescence and adolescence
   a. The child experiences intimate, dependent, same-sex relationships
   b. Dependent heterosexual relationships appear
   c. Independence from parents increases
   d. The child balances parental demands and peer group pressure
4. Young adulthood
   a. Interdependent relationships form
   b. The young adult makes independent decisions
   c. Occupational plans are implemented
   d. Dependent and independent behaviors are balanced
   e. Sensitivity to and acceptance of feelings and needs of the self and others increase
   f. Interpersonal relationships are characterized by mutuality

5. Middle adulthood
   a. Independence is fostered in others, such as children
   b. Self-reliance increases
   c. Interdependent relationship with children is established
6. Late adulthood
   a. The adult experiences and deals with losses
   b. New relationships develop
   c. Cultural contributions continue or increase
   d. As much independence as possible is retained, but increased dependence is accepted

♦ II. Personality disorders

A. General characteristics
   1. Maladaptive social responses
   2. Impaired social functioning
   3. Limited insight (and does not see a need to change behavior)
   4. Risky behaviors
   5. Troubles with legal system

B. Predisposing factors
   1. Developmental factors
      a. Any unaccomplished developmental task
      b. Disrupted relationship with the mothering person
   2. Family communication factors
      a. Disruptive relationships manifested in symptomatic behavior of one member
      b. Deviant behavior when the family is highly stressed
      c. Closed family system that discourages relationships with others
   3. Sociocultural factors
      a. Mores against casual acquaintances
      b. Mobility that contributes to transient friendships
      c. Social isolation, especially among elderly, handicapped, and chronically ill persons
      d. Romanticization of heterosexual relationships
   4. Neurobiological factors
      a. Studies of twins show a genetic vulnerability
      b. Difficult to discern affects of environment, parental roles, and genetics in studies of twins
   5. Biological factors
      a. Inconsistent evidence on role of neurotransmitters
      b. No identified biological cause

6. Child abuse
   a. High rate of early childhood traumas
   b. 67 to 86% have experienced sexual abuse
   c. 46 to 71% have experienced physical abuse

C. Treatment modalities
   1. Behavior modification
   2. COGNITIVE THERAPY
   3. Individual psychotherapy
   4. Milieu therapy
   5. Psychoeducation
   6. Psychopharmacology
      a. Antianxiety medications
      b. Antimanic medications
      c. Antidepressants
      d. Neuroleptics

◆ III. Dependency and helplessness

A. Nursing assessment
   1. Fear and anxiety
   2. Hypersensitivity to potential rejection
   3. Passive relinquishing of control
   4. Indirect RESISTANCE to occupational and social performance
   5. Clinging, demanding behavior
   6. Low self-esteem
   7. Exaggerated fear of losing control
   8. Preoccupation with control and power

B. Diagnoses
   1. Related *DSM-IV* medical diagnoses disorder
      a. Avoidant personality disorder
      b. Dependent personality disorder
      c. Obsessive-compulsive personality disorder
      d. Passive-aggressive personality disorder
   2. Related primary NANDA nursing diagnoses
      a. Personal identity disturbance
      b. Self-esteem disturbance
      c. Impaired social interaction

C. Nursing interventions
   1. Anticipate the patient's needs before the patient demands attention
   2. Set realistic limits for the patient
   3. Help the patient manage anxiety
   4. Establish trust
   5. Teach the patient and family to express ideas and feelings assertively
      (See *Family of a patient with a personality disorder,* page 104)

TEACHING TIPS
Family of a patient with a personality disorder

Be sure to include the following topics in your teaching plan for the family of a patient with a personality disorder.
- General information about relatedness
- Predisposing factors
- Appropriate methods for expression of feelings
- Communication techniques
- Treatment regimens
- Follow-up therapy
- Need for compliance

6. Support the patient in accepting increased decision making
7. Clarify roles between staff and patient and between patient and family members

◆ IV. Suspiciousness

A. Nursing assessment
1. Distrust
2. Rigidity
3. Expectations of trickery or harm
4. Secretiveness
5. Guardedness
6. Jealousy
7. Overconcern with hidden motives
8. Hypersensitivity and hyperalertness
9. Distortions of reality
10. PROJECTION

B. Diagnosis
1. Related *DSM-IV* medical diagnosis: Paranoid personality disorder
2. Related primary NANDA nursing diagnosis
   a. Personal identity disturbance
   b. Impaired social interaction

C. Nursing interventions
1. Overcome the patient's lack of insight and rigidity of thoughts
2. Establish communication with the patient and provide FEEDBACK as needed
3. Reduce social isolation
4. Keep messages clear and consistent

5. Avoid pretense and deception
6. Provide CONSENSUAL VALIDATION; reinforcement and corroboration from others helps to reinforce actual perception of reality
7. Foster trust
8. Minimize anxiety
9. Provide a supportive environment
10. Respect privacy

◆ V. Withdrawal

A. Nursing assessment
1. Incapable of forming warm, tender relationships
2. Indifferent to praise, criticisms, and feelings of others
3. Reclusive
4. Vague about goals
5. Indecisive
6. Detached

B. Diagnosis
1. Related *DSM-IV* medical diagnoses
   a. Schizoid personality disorder
   b. Schizotypal personality disorder
2. Related primary NANDA nursing diagnoses
   a. Personal identity disturbance
   b. Self-esteem disturbance
   c. Impaired social interaction

C. Nursing interventions
1. Attend to basic daily needs
2. Establish therapeutic interpersonal communication
3. Encourage social interactions with others
4. Establish realistic goals
5. Use consistent approaches

◆ VI. Impulsivity and manipulation

A. Nursing assessment
1. Inability to form significant loyalties or close, lasting relationships
2. Selfishness
3. Inability to delay gratification
4. Superficial charm and above-average intelligence
5. Unreliability
6. Insincerity
7. Lack of remorse, shame, guilt, or anxiety except under external stress
8. Inadequate motivation
9. Poor judgment
10. Failure to learn by experience

11. Egocentricity
12. Specific loss of insight
13. Failure to follow a life plan
14. Inability to tolerate frustration
15. Manipulativeness

B. Diagnoses
1. Related *DSM-IV* medical diagnoses
   a. Antisocial personality disorder
   b. Borderline personality disorder
   c. Histrionic personality disorder
   d. Narcissistic personality disorder
2. Related primary NANDA nursing diagnoses
   a. Personal identity disturbance
   b. Self-esteem disturbance
   c. Risk for self-mutilation
   d. Impaired social interaction
   e. Risk for violence

C. Nursing interventions
1. Overcome lack of motivation to change
2. Provide model of mature behavior
3. Assist in developing positive relationships
4. Convey concern and interest
5. Assist with problem solving
6. Encourage fewer acting-out behaviors
7. Facilitate verbal communication
8. Support patient's developmental growth
9. Anticipate and deal with depression
10. Set limits on manipulative behavior; this reinforces guidelines for behavior and provides structure and reliability
11. Assist patient in controlling personal anger and resentment

CLINICAL ALERT

POINTS TO REMEMBER

♦ Altered patterns of social relatedness are functional disturbances of personality.

♦ Personality disorders are lifelong behavior patterns that are acceptable to the individual but that create conflict with others.

♦ A combination of predisposing factors contributes to the development of personality disorders.

♦ Treatment is difficult because patients with personality disorders lack motivation to change.

◆ Nursing interventions for patients with personality disorders require self-awareness and action rather than reaction.

STUDY QUESTIONS

◆ To evaluate your understanding of this chapter, answer the following questions in the space provided; then compare your responses with the correct answers in Appendix B, page 172.

1. What are the characteristics of healthy interpersonal relationships? _____

_____

_____

2. Which steps does a young adult take in developing relatedness? _____

_____

_____

3. What can a nurse do if a patient experiences dependency and helplessness?

_____

_____

4. What is the key characteristic of a patient experiencing suspiciousness? ___

_____

_____

5. Which treatment modalities can a nurse use for a patient with a personality disorder? _____

_____

_____

CRITICAL THINKING AND APPLICATION EXERCISES

1. Research the *DSM-IV* for diagnostic criteria for personality disorders. Summarize the criteria for each type.

2. Review a patient's development of relatedness.

3. Observe a psychotherapy session. Prepare an oral presentation of your observations.

4. Care for a patient with a personality disorder. Develop a plan of care including follow-up.

CHAPTER

Psychoactive Substance Abuse

LEARNING OBJECTIVES

After studying this chapter, you should be able to:

♦ Identify five patterns of substance use and behavioral patterns of substance abusers.

♦ Discuss six predisposing factors of substance abuse.

♦ Identify the major categories of abused substances.

♦ Formulate individual nursing diagnoses appropriate for substance abuse disorders.

♦ Develop a nursing care plan for patients in the acute and rehabilitative phases of substance abuse.

CHAPTER OVERVIEW

Psychoactive substance abuse is a growing problem in society. It is believed that certain biological, psychological, and sociocultural factors predispose a person to substance abuse. Nursing care for a substance abuser requires a thorough assessment to determine which substance is being abused. Nursing care during the acute phase focuses on maintaining the patient's vital functions and safety. During rehabilitation, the nurse helps the patient focus on the problem of substance abuse and on alternative methods of dealing with stress. The nurse helps the patient focus on ways to achieve recovery and stay drug free.

♦ I. Overview of use and abuse

A. Terminology
 1. Substance abuse
  a. Continued use that interferes with the individual's biological, psychological, or sociocultural functioning
  b. A pervasive disorder
  c. Use that differs from approved medical or social patterns
 2. Substance dependence
  a. Considered a disease
  b. May have physical problems
  c. Serious disruption in social functioning
 3. Addiction
  a. Preoccupation with compulsive use
  b. Preoccupation with securing supply
  c. Tendency to renewed addiction after withdrawal
  d. Used interchangeably with the term "dependence"
 4. Physical dependence
  a. Body develops biological need for substance
  b. Tolerance and withdrawal symptoms develop
  c. Biological need can occur apart from dependence
 5. Withdrawal symptoms
  a. Occur when level of substance in body decreases
  b. Are a sign of physical dependence
 6. Tolerance
  a. Occurs when an increased amount of substance is needed to produce the same effect
  b. Is a sign of physical dependence

B. Patterns of substance use
 1. Experimental
 2. Recreational
 3. Circumstantial
  a. Used to cope with life's problems
  b. Carries potential for abuse
 4. Intensified
  a. Heavy, frequent use
  b. Abuse
 5. Compulsive
  a. High frequency
  b. High intensity
  c. Abuse
  d. Dependence

C. Prevalence
  1. Abuse occurs in all socioeconomic groups
  2. 90% of young adult population has tried alcohol
  3. Alcohol causes 50% of fatal auto accidents
  4. About 25% of all hospitalizations are alcohol related
  5. Approximately 12 million alcoholics live in the United States
  6. Men have higher addiction rates than women
  7. About 5% of U.S. population experiences drug abuse
  8. Fetal alcohol effects are a primary cause of mental retardation
  9. More women abuse prescription drugs

D. Predisposing factors
  1. Biological
    a. Familial tendency
    b. Possible genetic abnormality or inherited sensitivity
    c. Changes in neurotransmitters
  2. Psychological
    a. No addictive personality has been identified
    b. A link between abuse and depression as well as anxiety has been observed
    c. A link between abuse and certain personalities, such as antisocial and dependent, has been observed
  3. Sociocultural factors
    a. Use is influenced by nationality and ethnicity
    b. Religious sanctions influence use
    c. Alcohol use is more socially accepted than drug use, especially by men
  4. Learning theory
    a. Reflex response aimed at reducing anxiety
    b. Peer and parental modeling
    c. Positive reinforcement provided by drugs
    d. Continuation of abuse to avoid withdrawal symptoms
  5. Disease model
    a. Chronic, progressive disorder, which is potentially fatal
    b. Inherited predisposition
    c. Use of substance triggers the disease

E. Behavioral patterns
  1. Dysfunctional anger
  2. Manipulation
    a. Attempts to meet needs by influencing others
    b. Typically follows negative pattern of interaction
    c. Deceives others
    d. Makes others feel used, powerless, and angry

3. Impulsiveness
   a. Directs behaviors toward immediate gratification
   b. Acts abruptly
   c. May be active or passive
   d. Uses impulses to avoid conscious feelings of guilt and anger
4. Avoidance
   a. Facilitates an escape from anxiety associated with relatedness
   b. Is characterized by running away or emotional distancing
   c. Used to exert control over situations
5. Grandiosity
   a. Exalted or superior state
   b. Denial and rationalization of the consequences of behavior
   c. Commonly manifested by an unshakable belief in personal clever-
      ness

F. Commonly abused drugs
   1. Alcohol
   2. Stimulants
      a. Amphetamines
      b. Cocaine
      c. Caffeine
   3. Opiates and related analgesics
      a. Heroin
      b. Morphine
      c. Codeine
      d. Opium
      e. Methadone
      f. Hallucinogens
      g. Phencyclidine (PCP)
      h. Meperidine
   4. Depressants
      a. Alcohol
      b. Barbiturates
      c. Benzodiazepines
      d. Marijuana
   5. Inhalants
      a. Glue
      b. Cleaning solutions
      c. Nail polish remover
      d. Aerosols
      e. Petroleum products
      f. Paint thinners
   6. Designer drugs
      a. Variations of heroin, cocaine, and PCP
      b. China white

G. Treatment modalities
1. Behavior modification
2. Group therapy
3. Individual therapy
4. Social support systems
   a. Employee assistance programs
   b. Family counseling
   c. Halfway houses
   d. Self-help groups (such as Alcoholics Anonymous and Synanon)
5. Pharmacology
   a. Antabuse
   b. Methadone maintenance

♦ II. Alcohol abuse

A. General information
1. Alcohol is a sedative but creates a feeling of euphoria
2. Sedation increases as amount ingested increases
3. Characteristic behaviors are categorized into phases

B. Phases
1. Pre-alcoholic phase
   a. Use of alcohol to relax
   b. Increased tolerance
2. Early alcoholic phase
   a. Sneaking of drinks
   b. Denial of drinking
   c. Blackouts
   d. Increasing dependence
   e. Feelings of guilt
3. Crucial phase
   a. Loss of control over drinking
   b. Aggressive behavior
   c. Blaming of others for altered relationships
   d. Withdrawal symptoms, such as tremors
   e. Loss of other interests
   f. Problems with work and money
   g. Early morning drinking
   h. Decreased tolerance
4. Chronic phase
   a. Indulgence in unplanned sprees and lengthy intoxications
   b. Solitary drinking
   c. Physical complications
   d. Impaired thinking

     e. No more alibis

     f. Admission of defeat

  5. Rehabilitation

     a. Desires help

     b. Learns alcoholism is an illness

     c. Stops drinking

     d. Begins healthy thinking

     e. Develops support system

     f. Identifies hope for new way of life

  6. Recovery

     a. New interests

     b. New circle of friends

     c. Contentment in sobriety

     d. Natural rest and sleep patterns

     e. Increased emotional control

C. Nursing assessment

  1. Physiologic consequences

     a. Blackouts

     b. Pathologic intoxication

     c. Alcohol WITHDRAWAL SYNDROME

     d. Acute alcoholic hallucinosis

     e. Wernicke's syndrome

     f. Korsakoff's syndrome

     g. Alcoholic paranoia

     h. Liver damage

     i. Gout symptoms

     j. Alcoholic hepatitis

     k. Alcoholic cirrhosis

     l. Gastritis

     m. Gastric ulcers

     n. Pancreatitis

     o. Malnutrition

     p. Alcoholic cardiomyopathy

     q. Muscular myopathy

     r. Adrenocortical insufficiency

     s. Erection problems

  2. Withdrawal behavior

     a. Begins shortly after drinking stops

     b. Lasts 5 to 7 days

     c. Signaled by anxiety, anorexia, insomnia, tremors, hyperalertness, mild disorientation

     d. May include alcoholic hallucinosis (auditory hallucinations lasting for several hours), alcohol withdrawal delirium, and generalized motor seizures

D. Diagnoses
   1. Related *DSM-IV* medical diagnoses
      a. Alcohol dependence
      b. Alcohol abuse
      c. Alcohol intoxication
      d. Alcohol withdrawal
   2. Primary NANDA nursing diagnoses
      a. Ineffective individual coping
      b. Sensory or perceptual alteration
      c. Altered thought processes

**CLINICAL
ALERT**

E. Nursing implementation
   1. Acute stage
      a. Withdrawal
         (1) Monitor vital signs
         (2) Observe for signs of seizures and impending alcohol withdrawal syndrome
      b. Inadequate food and fluid intake
         (1) Provide high-protein diet
         (2) Provide mineral and vitamin supplements
         (3) Record fluid intake and output
         (4) Test urine for specific gravity and stool for blood
         (5) Encourage fluid intake
      c. Risk of self-injury
         (1) Provide supervision
         (2) Remove potentially harmful items
         (3) Reduce anxiety
      d. Self-care deficit
         (1) Assist with personal care
         (2) Delay unnecessary procedures
      e. Need for rest and relaxation
         (1) Avoid sudden approaches
         (2) Explain reasons for all tests and procedures
         (3) Provide measures to induce sleep
      f. Anxiety
         (1) Provide antianxiety drugs, as ordered
         (2) Explain reasons for all tests and procedures
         (3) Orient patient to reality
         (4) Encourage patient to vent fear and anger
   2. Rehabilitation
      a. Denial of illness
         (1) Help patient accept that drinking must stop
         (2) Confront denial and manipulation

      b. Failure of patient to understand the disease
        (1) Educate the patient about alcoholism
        (2) Teach the effects of abuse
      c. Low self-esteem
        (1) Engage patient in tasks that lead to success
        (2) Explore areas of competence
        (3) Express hope of arresting alcoholism
      d. Loneliness
        (1) Provide positive interpersonal experiences
        (2) Help patient express needs directly
        (3) Identify ways of alleviating loneliness
      e. Low tolerance for frustration
        (1) Explore methods of relieving tension and anxiety
        (2) Assist in developing constructive coping skills
      f. Possibility of relapse
        (1) Complete discharge planning
        (2) Inform patient of available support systems

♦ III. Drug abuse

A. General information
  1. Use of multiple substances is increasing
  2. Choice of substance is influenced by availability and exposure
  3. Health care professionals tend to abuse prescription drugs

B. Physiologic consequences of drug abuse
  1. Circulatory and respiratory complications
    a. Bacterial endocarditis
    b. Gangrene
    c. Thrombophlebitis
    d. Sclerosing of veins
    e. Intracranial hemorrhage
    f. Pulmonary embolism
    g. Respiratory infections
    h. Tuberculosis
    i. Pulmonary abscesses
    j. Acquired immunodeficiency syndrome
  2. Hepatic complications
  3. Gastrointestinal complications
    a. Severe and rapid weight loss
    b. Vitamin deficiencies
    c. Severe constipation
    d. Hemorrhoids

4. Integumentary complications
   a. Scarring
   b. Abscesses
   c. Cellulitis
   d. Ulcerations
5. Muscular complications
   a. Fibrosing myopathy
   b. Chronic muscle damage
6. Other complications
   a. Tetanus
   b. Eye emboli
   c. Traumatic injury

C. Nursing assessment
1. Opiate abuse
   a. Mental and physical deterioration
   b. Inability to function productively
   c. Pursuit of illegal behavior
   d. Rapidly developed tolerance
   e. Decreased response to pain
   f. Respiratory depression
   g. Nausea
   h. Constriction of pupils
   i. Drowsiness
   j. Depressed pituitary functioning
   k. Slowed peristalsis
   l. Constipation
   m. Euphoria
   n. Apathy
   o. Detachment from reality
   p. Impaired judgment
   q. Uncomfortable (but not life-threatening) withdrawal symptoms
   r. Psychological addiction
   s. Physical dependence
2. Stimulant abuse
   a. Alertness
   b. Hyperactivity
   c. Irritability
   d. Insomnia
   e. Anorexia
   f. Weight loss
   g. Tachycardia
   h. Hypertension
   i. Psychological dependence
   j. Rapidly developed tolerance (within hours or days)

      k. Panic reactions
      l. Paranoid delusions
     m. Suspicion
  3. Depressant abuse
      a. Lethargy
      b. Sleepiness
      c. Respiratory depression
      d. Circulatory depression
      e. Tolerance
      f. Withdrawal symptoms with abrupt cessation
      g. Temporary psychoses
  4. Hallucinogen abuse
      a. Intensified sensory experiences
      b. Distortion of time and space
      c. Absence of addiction
      d. Impaired judgment
      e. Delusions
      f. Hallucinations
      g. Flashbacks
      h. Antisocial behaviors
  5. Marijuana abuse
      a. Altered state of awareness
      b. Relaxation
      c. Mild euphoria
      d. Slowed reflexes
      e. Reduced inhibitions
      f. Apathy
      g. Lack of motivation
      h. Fine tremors
      i. Decreased muscle strength
      j. Decreased coordination
      k. Absence of tolerance
      l. Absence of physical dependence
  6. Inhalant abuse
      a. Euphoria
      b. Decreased inhibition
      c. Misperceptions or illusions
      d. Cloudiness of thought
      e. Drowsiness
      f. Rapidly developed tolerance
      g. Absence of withdrawal symptoms

D. Diagnoses
  1. Related *DSM-IV* medical diagnoses
    a. Amphetamine (substance) abuse
    b. (Substance) dependence
    c. (Substance) intoxication
    d. (Substance) withdrawal
    e. Polysubstance dependence
  2. Primary NANDA nursing diagnoses
    a. Ineffective individual coping
    b. Sensory or perceptual alteration
    c. Altered thought processes

E. Nursing implementation
  1. Acute drug reactions (See *Immediate care for a patient with cocaine intoxication*)
    a. Decreased circulatory and respiratory function
      (1) Monitor vital signs and neurologic reflex responses
      (2) Suction as necessary
      (3) Monitor for possible cardiopulmonary resuscitation
    b. Impending withdrawal
      (1) Assess the current stage of withdrawal
      (2) Administer medications, as ordered
      (3) Approach the patient calmly; avoid touching the patient; patient may be in a heightened state of alertness
      (4) Limit visitors
    c. Potential for self-injury
      (1) Restrain patient as needed
      (2) Remove harmful objects
      (3) Monitor suicidal behavior
    d. Panic and flashback reactions
      (1) Remain with patient
      (2) Encourage expression of feelings
      (3) Provide reassurance by orienting patient to reality
      (4) Do not support delusions or hallucinations
    e. Poor nutritional status
      (1) Administer skin care
      (2) Record intake and output
      (3) Provide small, frequent feedings
      (4) Administer I.V. solutions as prescribed
  2. Drug rehabilitation
    a. Recognize denial of the illness
    b. Focus on the problem of substance abuse
    c. Avoid the patient's attempts to focus only on external problems
    d. Identify the projection of blame or defensiveness
    e. Avoid discussions of unanswerable questions

CLINICAL ALERT

DECISION TREE

Immediate care for a patient with cocaine intoxication

The decision tree below highlights the major care activities for a patient with acute cocaine intoxication.

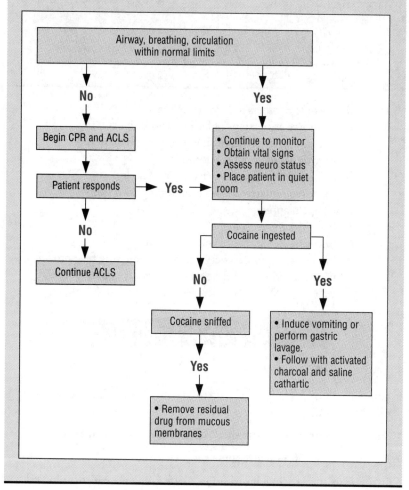

3. Lack of knowledge about consequences of drug use
   a. Provide factual information
   b. Dispel myths
4. Avoidance of responsibility
   a. Encourage the patient to identify behaviors that cause difficulties
   b. Do not allow the patient to rationalize or to blame others
   c. Refocus on the patient's problems

TEACHING TIPS
Patient with substance abuse problems

Be sure to include the following topics in your teaching plan for the patient who is a substance abuser and his family.
• Problems associated with substance abuse
• Facts versus myths
• Positive reinforcement
• Alternative coping mechanisms
• Support groups
• Compliance and follow-up

     d. Encourage others to provide feedback
     e. Reinforce expressions of feelings and insights
     f. Encourage verbal expression of anger and depression
     g. Provide a structured environment
     h. Prepare the patient for a change in lifestyle
     i. Discuss alternative methods of dealing with stress
  5. Discharge planning
     a. Identify support systems
     b. Encourage compliance with treatment
     c. Explore goals for recovery and for staying drug free; provide patient education (See *Patient with substance abuse problems*)

POINTS TO REMEMBER

◆ Any drug can be misused.

◆ Substance abuse is a behavioral pattern that involves all aspects of the patient's functioning.

◆ Substance abuse poses a major health problem in the United States.

◆ No simple cause of substance abuse has been identified or accepted.

◆ In the acute stage of drug intoxication, maintaining the patient's physical well-being takes priority.

STUDY QUESTIONS

To evaluate your understanding of this chapter, answer the following questions in the space provided; then compare your responses with the correct answers in Appendix B, pages 172 and 173.

1. Which behaviors might a nurse observe in a substance abuser?_____

_____

_____

2. What are three predisposing psychological factors associated with substance abuse? _____

_____

_____

3. Which behaviors are associated with each phase of alcoholism? _____

_____

_____

4. How can the nurse intervene during alcohol withdrawal? _____

_____

_____

5. What are three problems that the nurse may have to confront during the rehabilitative stage of alcoholism? _____

_____

_____

6. If a patient is suspected of inhalant abuse, which behaviors might be exhibited? _____

_____

_____

7. Which problems should a nurse anticipate during a patient's acute drug reaction?_____

_____

_____

8. How should a nurse handle a patient's denial during drug rehabilitation? __

_____

_____

CRITICAL THINKING AND APPLICATION EXERCISES

1. Research the various types of stimulants available. Create a table listing the street name, routes, duration, signs and symptoms of use and withdrawal.

2. Prepare a presentation for junior high school students about the effects of substance abuse.

3. Develop a plan of care from admission through discharge for a patient with substance abuse. Include plans for education and follow-up.

CHAPTER

13

Disorders Associated with Anger and Violence

LEARNING OBJECTIVES

After studying this chapter, you should be able to:

♦ Differentiate between anger, violence and abuse.

♦ Formulate individual nursing diagnoses for patients experiencing anger and aggressive behavior.

♦ Formulate individual nursing diagnoses for violent offenders.

♦ Formulate individual nursing diagnoses for victims of abuse.

♦ Name at least six factors that increase one's potential for violence.

♦ Develop nursing care plans for intervening with the angry or the verbally or physically aggressive patient.

♦ Identify five characteristics of a violent family system.

♦ Identify nursing interventions for patients who have been physically abused.

♦ Identify nursing interventions for patients who have been sexually abused.

CHAPTER OVERVIEW

Disorders associated with anger and violence take many forms, span all socio-economic and cultural groups, and have devastating consequences. Crucial to the management of these disorders is an understanding of the underlying characteristics, etiologies, and responses and cues. A thorough assessment provides the foundation for individual interventions aimed at improving control and preventing harm. A nursing self-assessment about one's own feelings and responses is essential for effective outcomes.

♦ I. Anger

A. Description
1. Characteristics
   a. Serves as a natural adaptation to disruption
   b. Is characterized by tension
   c. Occurs in response to anxiety from a perceived threat
   d. Ranges from mild annoyance to rage or fury
   e. Is related to a fear of rejection
2. Functional anger
   a. Energizes behavior to avoid anxiety
   b. Characterizes a healthy relationship
   c. Can project a positive self-concept
   d. Serves as an ego defense; more effective than anxiety
   e. Gives the person a sense of control
   f. Indicates a need for more effective coping behaviors
   g. Provides immediate relief
3. Dysfunctional anger
   a. Arises when early conflicts are reenacted
   b. Becomes a source of tension. Is cyclical, stemming from or resulting in:
      (1) Unresolved anxiety and anger
      (2) Offensive behaviors
      (3) Powerlessness in others
      (4) Angry response or rejection by others
B. Modes of expression
1. External
   a. Constructive criticism
   b. AGGRESSION

2. Internal
   a. Nonassertiveness
   b. Self-destruction
3. Direct
4. Indirect
   a. Passivity
   b. Manipulation
   c. Acting-out behavior
   d. Displaced onto safe objects
5. Precipitating stressors
   a. Individual
   b. External or internal threatening event

C. Nursing assessment
   1. Physical responses associated with anger (resulting from action of the autonomic nervous system in response to epinephrine secretion)
      a. Increased blood pressure
      b. Tachycardia
      c. Altered blood composition
      d. Increased salivation
      e. Nausea
      f. Increased hydrochloric acid secretion
      g. Decreased gastric peristalsis
      h. Increased alertness and muscle tension
      i. Accelerated reflexes
      j. Increased urination
      k. Dilated pupils
      l. Flushed face
      m. Sweating
   2. Emotional responses associated with anger
      a. Discomfort
      b. Powerlessness
      c. Annoyance
      d. Frustration
      e. Resentment
      f. Belligerence
      g. Rage
      h. Humiliation
      i. Defensiveness
      j. Inadequacy
      k. Depression
      l. HOSTILITY
      m. Guilt
      n. Acting-out behavior

3. Intellectual responses associated with anger
   a. Sarcasm
   b. Argumentativeness
   c. Fault finding
   d. Domination
   e. Belittling
   f. Scolding
   g. Blaming
   h. Forgetfulness
   i. Repetitive thoughts
   j. RUMINATION
   k. Projection
   l. Ridicule
4. Social responses associated with anger
   a. Withdrawal
   b. Alienation
   c. Rejection
   d. Teasing
   e. Humor
   f. Violence
   g. Poor self-concept
   h. Demand making
   i. Intimidation
   j. Overactivity
   k. Hypersensitivity
   l. Substance abuse
5. Spiritual responses associated with anger
   a. Omnipotence
   b. Self-righteousness
   c. Self-doubt
   d. Demoralization
   e. Sinfulness
   f. Blocked creativity

D. Nursing planning and implementation
   1. Outcomes
      a. The patient will establish a hierarchy of behaviors
      b. The patient will reinforce mastery and self-control
      c. The patient will learn appropriate expression of anger
   2. Interventions
      a. Provide constructive outlets, protection, and control
      b. Remain with the patient, and do not become defensive
      c. Set and enforce appropriate limits

    d. Reduce sources of anxiety

    e. Acknowledge the patient's anger, and help the patient recognize those feelings; acknowledgement and validation help to foster trust and can help encourage the patient to describe angry feelings and to explore reasons for the anger

    f. Clarify misunderstandings

    g. Communicate that anger is acceptable

    h. Help the patient use assertive behaviors

    i. Enhance the patient's self-esteem

    j. Monitor personal anxiety level

    k. Prevent violence

E. Evaluation
1. Behavioral changes
2. Subjective responses of the patient
3. Appropriateness of expressions of anger
4. Use of assertive behaviors
5. Successful problem solving

◆ II. Aggression and violence

A. Description
1. Characteristics
    a. Aggression is a natural drive
    (1) Is destructive when uncontrolled
    (2) Evokes a defensive response
    (3) Can be instrumental or hostile
    (4) Can be direct or indirect
    (5) Can be a precursor of violence
    (6) Is often a cover up for a lack of self-confidence
    b. Violence carries physical, emotional, or moral force
    (1) Poses a threat to others and arouses their fears
    (2) Creates anxiety in victims
    (3) Is displayed deliberately or follows a loss of control over aggressive impulses
2. Theories of aggression
    a. Psychoanalytic theory
    (1) Aggression is instinctual
    (2) The aggressor attempts to master personal inferiority
    b. Drive theory (frustration-aggression theory)
    (1) Frustration occurs when goal achievement is blocked; frustration leads to anger, anxiety, and aggression
    (2) This innate response can be inhibited

    c. Social learning theory (behavior basis)
      (1) Aggression is a learned behavior
      (2) The social environment instigates and reinforces aggression
      (3) Violence is a functional behavior designed to control others
    d. Need theory
      (1) Aggression is a method of communicating a need
      (2) Aggression (destructive behavior) is used when a need cannot be met through constructive behavior
    e. Stress adaptation theory
      (1) Any activity requiring a response generates stress
      (2) Stress carries the potential for violence
    f. Biochemical theory
      (1) The limbic system regulates aggressive behavior
      (2) A lesion of the hypothalamus and amygdala increases or decreases aggressive behavior
      (3) Release of norepinephrine by the adrenal medulla directly influences aggressive behavior
      (4) Increased blood levels of testosterone in males correlate with increased aggressiveness
      (5) Decreased progesterone blood levels in females correlate with increased hostility
      (6) Frontal lobe damage can lead to aggressive outbursts
      (7) Aggressive behavior may occur during or after seizure activity
    g. Sociocultural theory
      (1) Cultural norms define acceptable and unacceptable means of expressing aggression
      (2) Legal systems apply sanctions to violators of societal norms.
  3. Precipitating stressors
    a. Psychotic conditions and impaired thought processes
    b. Organic conditions
    c. Depression
    d. Disorders of impulse control; antisocial behavior
    e. Ineffective coping skills
    f. Dysfunctional family systems
    g. Disturbed roles within the family system
    h. Disturbed marital relationships
    i. Violent expressions of anger

B. Treatment modalities
  1. Crisis intervention
  2. Hospital emergency departments
  3. Individual counseling
  4. Behavior modification
  5. Social support systems
  6. Assertiveness training

TEACHING TIPS
Patient with aggression and violence

Be sure to include the following topics in your teaching plan when caring for a patient who is aggressive and violent.
- Definition and possible causes
- Treatment modalities
- Manifestations
- Methods to enhance self-control
- Alternative appropriate behaviors

---

      7. Victim group sessions
      8. Family therapy
      9. Spiritual counseling
   10. Patient education (See *Patient with aggression and violence*)
   11. Psychopharmacology
      a. Antianxiety and sedative-hypnotics for acute agitation
      b. Antidepressants and lithium to control moods
      c. Antipsychotics
   12. Substance abuse treatment
  C. Nursing assessment
    1. Behavioral cues
      a. Change in usual behavior
      b. Glaring
      c. Restlessness
      d. Rigid posture
      e. Clenched hands
      f. Ingestion of alcohol or drugs
      g. Overt, aggressive actions
      h. Physical withdrawal
      i. Noncompliance
      j. Overreaction
      k. Hostile threats
      l. Talk of past violent acts
      m. Argumentativeness
      n. Profanity
      o. Abusive belittling
      p. Somatic complaint or preoccupation
      q. Invading others' space
      r. Staring

2. Cognitive cues
   a. Inability to express feelings
   b. Repetitive demands and complaints
   c. Disorientation
   d. Inability to focus attention
   e. Hallucinations or delusions
   f. Paranoid ideas or suspicions

D. Diagnoses
   1. Related *DSM-IV* medical diagnoses
      a. Conduct disorder
      b. Anxiety disorder
      c. Intermittent explosive disorder
      d. Impulse control not otherwise specified
   2. Primary NANDA diagnostic categories
      a. Ineffective individual coping
      b. Risk for violence: self-directed or directed at others
      c. Anxiety

E. Nursing planning and implementation
   1. Outcomes
      a. The patient will not experience further loss of control
      b. The patient will demonstrate a restoration of self-control
      c. Patient will not harm self or others
   2. Interventions for a potentially violent patient
      a. Be aware of precursive signs
      b. Ask other patients or visitors to leave the area
      c. Maintain a reasonable physical distance from the patient; close proximity invades the patient's space, is threatening to him, and may escalate his anger and violence
      d. Explain to the patient all actions that the staff will carry out
      e. Offer reassurance of safety
      f. Remove objects that could be used destructively
      g. Seek assistance from other health care personnel, if needed
      h. Provide sedation, if required and prescribed
      i. Help the patient distinguish among thoughts, feelings, and behaviors
      j. Explore alternative behaviors
      k. Encourage the patient to consider the consequences of violent behavior
      l. Set firm limits on the patient's behavior
   3. Interventions for a verbally aggressive patient
      a. Remain with the patient
      b. Do not become angry or defensive
      c. Be aware of personal anxiety level; patient may sense the nurse's increasing level which may escalate the situation

CLINICAL ALERT

CLINICAL ALERT

    d. Provide consistent expectations and guidelines for the patient's self-control

    e. Acknowledge the patient's anger, and state that anger is an acceptable feeling

    f. Explore the precipitating threat or frustration

    g. Promote insight into the need for control

  4. Interventions for a physically aggressive patient

    a. Take precautions to ensure personal safety; do not attempt to handle the patient alone

    b. Approach the patient calmly and firmly

    c. Use short, concise statements

    d. Inform the patient of what is expected

    e. Provide medication

    f. Arrange for SECLUSION of the patient

    g. Use physical restraints as necessary

F. Evaluation

  1. Identify precipitating factors

  2. Evaluate effectiveness of techniques to diffuse a potentially violent patient

    a. Effectiveness of use of seclusion or restraints

    b. Patient's acknowledgment of improvement in ability to express anger constructively and maintain self-control

♦ III. Rape trauma

A. Description

  1. Characteristics

    a. Comprises verbal assaults, threats, intimidation, and physical force

    b. Occurs without the victim's consent

    c. Constitutes a traumatic event that serves as a precursor of crisis

    d. Rape is a crime of violence

    e. There is no typical victim

  2. Incidence

    a. Lack of accurate information on prevalence because assault victims typically are reluctant to report the assault

    b. Increase in reporting of sexual abuse of children, although experts say that most cases still go unreported

    c. Evidence that 40% to 60% of victims are raped by someone they know

  3. Motivations for sexual assault

    a. An act of aggression (it is not a sexual act)

    b. A means of gaining control

    c. A desire to humiliate, defile, or dominate the victim

  4. Reactions of rape victims

    a. Panic during the attack
    b. Humiliation, confusion, fear, and rage after the attack
    c. Long-term emotional effects (persist for several years)
      (1) Victimization and vulnerability
      (2) Degradation
      (3) Shame
      (4) Guilt
      (5) Self-blame
      (6) Wish for revenge

B. Treatment modalities for the victim
  1. Medical evaluation
  2. Group therapy
  3. Self-help groups

C. Assessment
  1. Behavioral characteristics
    a. Agitation
    b. Outward calmness
    c. Crying
    d. Nightmares
    e. Sleep problems
    f. Phobia
    g. Relationship difficulties
  2. Affective characteristics
    a. Shock
    b. Disbelief
    c. Fear
    d. Depression
    e. Feeling unclean and contaminated
    f. Alienation
    g. Anger
  3. Cognitive characteristics
    a. Depersonalization
    b. Denial
    c. Difficulty making decisions
    d. Self-blame
    e. Obsessional thoughts
    f. Flashbacks
    g. Violent dreams
    h. Social withdrawal
  4. Physiologic characteristics
    a. Physical injury
    b. Bleeding or trauma to vital organs
    c. Sore and swollen vagina or rectum

d. Tearing of vaginal or rectal wall
e. Traumatized throat
f. Pregnancy
g. Sexually transmitted disease
h. Sexual dysfunction

D. Diagnoses
1. Related *DSM-IV* medical diagnoses
   a. Post-traumatic stress disorder
   b. Sexual abuse
   c. Physical abuse
2. Primary NANDA nursing diagnoses
   a. Rape-trauma syndrome
   b. Rape-trauma syndrome: Compound reaction
   c. Rape-trauma syndrome: Silent reaction

E. Nursing planning and implementation
1. Outcomes
   a. Patient will regain emotional control and return to previous level of functioning
   b. Patient will verbalize rediscovery of self-respect and dignity

CLINICAL ALERT

2. Interventions
   a. Follow institutional protocols for notifying the police and collecting evidence of sexual assault; this ensures reliability of evidence should prosecution be pursued
      (1) Record the date, the time, and the officer's name
      (2) Collect evidence (clothing, fingernail scrapings, semen) in the presence of a witness, label the evidence carefully, and document findings
   b. Perform a thorough assessment and physical examination
      (1) Observe the patient's general appearance; measure and record vital signs
      (2) Obtain a medical history, including the rape
      (3) Note signs of vaginal or anal bleeding, bruises, lacerations, and redness; measure the size and note the location of injuries
      (4) Obtain vaginal swabs and smears
      (5) Advise the patient of a 6-week follow-up examination to rule out sexually transmitted diseases
      (6) Document findings
      (7) If needed, obtain consent for photographs
   c. Take steps to support the patient emotionally
      (1) Pursue CRISIS INTERVENTION when warranted, such as in rape-trauma syndrome
      (2) Provide a private, quiet environment where the patient can feel safe and think clearly

(3) Encourage the patient to discuss the assault, if able
(4) Initially, focus on the patient's immediate feelings (such as guilt, shame, or ambivalence); then discuss other issues, such as the patient's options, possible legal procedures, and counseling
(5) Refer the patient for continuing counseling, if desired

F. Evaluation
1. Patient's responses to supportive counseling
2. Patient's resolution of crisis

♦ IV. Family violence and abuse

A. Description
1. Etiologic theories
   a. Psychodynamic theory
      (1) Deprivation of nurturance in childhood
      (2) Victim of physical or sexual abuse as a child
      (3) Antisocial behavior
      (4) Mental illness
   b. Social learning theory
      (1) Lack of healthy role models for parenting and problem solving
      (2) A learned response; typically evident in many generations of the same family
   c. Environmental stress theory
      (1) Stress (such as from unemployment or poverty) that triggers abuse
      (2) Societal factors that promote and maintain violent expression
      (3) Inequity between stronger and weaker persons
      (4) Socialization that teaches women and children to be subservient
   d. Family systems theory
      (1) Faulty structure in family system
      (2) Inability of family members to define themselves as individuals apart from the family
      (3) Conflict within the family system
2. Categories of family violence
   a. Physical abuse
      (1) Slapping, kicking, or punching
      (2) Hitting or whipping with a blunt instrument
      (3) Pulling hair
      (4) Inflicting burns
      (5) Throwing an individual
      (6) Choking or gagging
      (7) Tying to a bed, chair, or crib
      (8) Locking in a closet or room for an extended period
      (9) Attempting to drown or hang

    b. Neglect
       (1) Failure to provide food, bed, shelter, clothing, health care, or sensory stimulation or to meet hygiene needs
       (2) Inability or refusal to protect against accidents or otherwise ensure safety
    c. Psychological unavailability
       (1) Ignorance of an individual's needs
       (2) Failure to provide sufficient affection or warmth
       (3) Inability to appreciate accomplishment or competence
       (4) Failure to respect privacy, preferences, or opinions
       (5) Unwillingness to share pleasant experiences or social events
    d. Verbal hostility
       (1) Name calling
       (2) Use of obscenities
       (3) Severe criticism
       (4) Use of humiliation and shame
       (5) Threats
    e. Sexual abuse
       (1) Rape
       (2) Sodomy
       (3) INCEST
       (4) EXHIBITIONISM (sometimes accompanied by masturbation)
3. Epidemiology of family violence
    a. Spouse abuse
       (1) Women are usually the victims; wife abuse is the most common cause of trauma in women
       (2) The problem spans all socioeconomic classes
       (3) 15% to 20% of homicides involve spouse abuse
    b. Child abuse
       (1) Few reliable statistics exist
       (2) The problem spans all socioeconomic classes
    c. Elder abuse
       (1) An estimated 10% of elderly adults are abused
       (2) The abuser is typically the elderly person's adult child
       (3) Elder abuse also occurs in institutions, such as nursing homes
4. Characteristics of violent families
    a. Multigenerational transmission
    b. Social isolation
    c. Use and abuse of power
    d. Alcohol and drug abuse
5. Treatment modalities
    a. CRISIS INTERVENTION
    b. Individual counseling
    c. Psychotherapy groups

    d. Self-help groups
    e. Family therapy
    f. Community support services

B. Nursing assessment
  1. Characteristics of the violent family system
    a. Closed boundaries
    b. Painful and desperate mood
    c. Competition for affection, caring, attention, and nurturance
    d. Inability of family members to define themselves as individuals apart from the family
    e. Inability to trust others
    f. Conflict within the family system
    g. Lack of impulse control and self-discipline
    h. Reduced capacity to delay gratification
    i. Focus on the present
    j. Inadequate task performance
    k. Mixed or double messages in communications
    l. Faulty perception of reality
    m. Imbalanced power ratio (one member has control over other members)
    n. Stereotyping of roles
  2. Characteristics of offenders
    a. Exhibits cyclical behavior
    b. Is immature and lacks self-control
    c. Displays insecurity
    d. Is dominant, rigid, and moralistic
    e. Shows aggressiveness
    f. Needs immediate gratification
    g. Lacks guilt
    h. Has symbiotic personality and poor interpersonal relationships
    i. Exhibits substance abuse
  3. Characteristics of abusing parent
    a. Is depressed
    b. Has unrealistic expectations of the child (as if the child were much older)
    c. Looks to children as a source of reassurance while projecting own problems onto the children
    d. Lacks confidence in parenting abilities, so feels children are the source of troubles
    e. Has hypochondriacal complaints
    f. Has a history of having been abused
  4. Spouse victim
    a. Displays ambivalence or fear
    b. Has low self-esteem, so feels responsible for provoking anger

    c. Rationalizes the abuse
    d. Is socially isolated
5. Child victim
    a. Runs away from home
    b. Displays age-inappropriate sexual behavior
    c. Is one whose age, sex, physical appearance, or personality may trigger conflict for the parent
    d. Shows ambivalence, depression, anxiety, fear
6. Elderly victim
    a. Is demanding and may act helpless or hopeless before the abuse
    b. May be belligerent and aggressive before the abuse
7. Physical symptoms
    a. Bruises
    b. Lacerations
    c. Broken bones
    d. Symptoms of anxiety and stress
    e. Chronic fatigue
    f. Old scars and bruises
    g. Bite marks
    h. Burns
    i. Blackened eyes
    j. Retarded growth or development in children
    k. Poor hygiene
8. Behavioral cues
    a. General
      (1) Inconsistent or irrational account of causes of injuries
      (2) Significant time lapse between injury and treatment
      (3) Family member's refusal to permit diagnostic tests; hasty exit from the examination room
      (4) Unwillingness of significant other to comfort the victim
    b. Cues related to all victims
      (1) Withdrawal or extreme aggression
      (2) Tendency to startle easily
      (3) Disturbed sleep patterns
      (4) Evasive comments about injury
      (5) Avoidance of eye contact
      (6) Vacant or frozen stare
      (7) Chronic lateness or truancy from job or school
      (8) Apology for seeking treatment
    c. Cues related to child victims
      (1) Wariness of adults
      (2) Rapid adaptation to hospital unit
      (3) Unwillingness to turn to family member or parents for support
      (4) Delinquent behavior

(5) Abnormal eating or drinking habits
(6) Excessive or absent crying
(7) Extreme fear of or total lack of respect for authority figures

C. Diagnoses
1. Related *DSM-IV* medical diagnoses
   a. Physical abuse of child
   b. Physical abuse of adult
   c. Sexual abuse of child
   d. Sexual abuse of adult
   e. Neglect
2. Primary NANDA nursing diagnoses
   a. Ineffective individual coping
   b. Ineffective family coping
   c. Altered parenting
   d. Self-esteem disturbance
   e. Risk for violence

D. Nursing planning and implementation
1. Outcomes
   a. Patient remains free from abuse
   b. Family members demonstrate enhanced communication
   c. Patient or family demonstrates appropriate expressions of anger
   d. Patient demonstrates improvement in parenting skills
2. Interventions
   a. For abused victim
      (1) Report abuse to authorities; it's the law
      (2) Ensure the patient's safety
      (3) Refer the patient and family to appropriate resources
      (4) Arrange for a medical examination
      (5) Collect evidence (such as the location and extent of injuries)
      (6) Offer anticipatory guidance and counseling
      (7) Explain legal procedures
      (8) Separate the victim from the offender
   b. For families
      (1) Teach effective communication skills
         (a) Negotiation
         (b) Problem solving
      (2) Identify methods for managing anger appropriately
         (a) Talk about anger as it occurs
         (b) Define limits and consequences of anger

    c. For abusive parents
       (1) Recognize current positive parenting skills
       (2) Assist to increase self-worth
       (3) Teach about normal growth and development
       (4) Identify solutions to specific problems in raising children

E. Evaluation
  1. Complete a nursing self-assessment
  2. Determine the effectiveness of nursing interventions in meeting the patient's physical care needs
  3. Ensure that the patient's medical record is complete and accurate
  4. Review involvement with community services and responses to support

POINTS TO REMEMBER

♦ Anger is a natural response to feelings of inadequacy and may be expressed overtly or covertly, externally or internally.

♦ Violence and assaultive behavior are unhealthy, destructive expressions of aggressive drive.

♦ Family abuse and violence span all socioeconomic classes and cultural groups.

♦ Sexual assault is an act of aggression.

♦ Violence is commonly a learned behavior that persists in many generations of the same family.

♦ Nurses should be aware of their own feelings and responses.

♦ Nursing goals and interventions must be individual to meet the patient's needs.

STUDY QUESTIONS

To evaluate your understanding of this chapter, answer the following questions in the space provided; then compare your responses to the correct answers in Appendix B, pages 173 and 174.

1. How does functional anger differ from dysfunctional anger? _____

_____

_____

2. What are two nursing care outcomes for a patient experiencing anger? _____

_____

_____

3. What are the characteristics of violence? _____

_____

_____

4. What are the major characteristics of a violent family system?_____

_____

_____

5. Which behavioral clues should a nurse look for when assessing a possible victim of child abuse? _____

_____

_____

6. What are three motivations for sexual assault? _____

_____

_____

7. What should the nurse do with evidence collected in a sexual assault case?

_____

_____

8. How should a nurse intervene with a physically aggressive patient?_____

_____

_____

CRITICAL THINKING AND APPLICATION EXERCISES

1. Perform a self-assessment about your feelings and behaviors when you're angry. Note how you respond to anger. Develop appropriate suggestions for change.

2. Review your health care institution's policy for handling rape-trauma evidence. Contact your local police department to find out how they handle evidence for trial.

3. Observe a community support group for family violence. Prepare an oral presentation describing your observations. Note the teaching methods used during the session(s).

4. Develop a plan of care from admission through discharge for a patient who has been abused. Be sure to include plans for education and follow-up.

CHAPTER

Cognitive Impairment Disorders

LEARNING OBJECTIVES

After studying this chapter, you should be able to:

♦ Identify behaviors associated with cognitive impairment disorders.

♦ Differentiate between delirium and dementia.

♦ Formulate nursing diagnoses for patients experiencing maladaptive cognitive responses.

♦ Develop nursing plans of care for patients experiencing delirium and dementia.

CHAPTER OVERVIEW

The cognitive impairment disorders DELIRIUM and DEMENTIA are commonly associated with the elderly. Thorough assessment is necessary to identify the cognitive, behavioral, affective, and physiologic characteristics of each. When caring for a patient with a cognitive impairment disorder, maintaining the patient's safety is the primary concern.

◆ I. Delirium

A. Description
   1. Acute onset usually lasting about 1 week
   2. Potentially reversible but life threatening if not treated
   3. Impaired cognition, perception, and behavior
   4. Often a sign of underlying medical problem in older patients
   5. Common in children and adults over 60 years old
   6. Caused by cerebral hypoxia, infection, drugs, metabolic disorders

B. Nursing assessment
   1. Behavioral characteristics
      a. Poor impulse control
      b. Altered psychomotor activity
         (1) Apathetic and withdrawn
         (2) Agitated and tremulous
         (3) Shifts between apathy and agitation
      c. Speech limited and dull, or pressured and loud
      d. Picking at bed linen and clothes
      e. Unable to complete tasks
      f. Bizarre, destructive behavior, worsens at night
   2. Affective characteristics
      a. Ranging from apathy to euphoria
      b. Emotionally labile
      c. Fear as predominant emotion
   3. Cognitive characteristics
      a. Disorganized thinking
      b. Rambling, bizarre, or incoherent speech
      c. Difficulty focusing attention
      d. Impaired decision making
      e. Easily distracted
      f. Recent memory impairment
      g. Disoriented (especially to time and place)
      h. Visual or auditory illusions
      i. Delusions
      j. Visual hallucinations
      k. Terrifying dreams
   4. Sociocultural characteristics
      a. Families are anxious and frightened
      b. Family members are unaware of how to respond
      c. Family's perception of events may be unclear
   5. Physiologic characteristics
      a. Disturbed sleep
      b. Increased cardiac rate
      c. Elevated blood pressure

      d. Flushed face
      e. Dilated pupils
      f. Sweating
      g. Altered respiratory depth or rhythm
      h. Tremors
      i. Generalized seizures

C. Diagnoses
    1. Related *DSM-IV* medical diagnoses
      a. Delirium due to a general medical condition
      b. Substance-induced delirium
      c. Delirium due to multiple etiologies
    2. Primary NANDA nursing diagnosis: Altered thought process

D. Nursing planning and implementation
    1. Outcomes
      a. Vary, depending on underlying physiologic cause
      b. Primary goal is to prevent permanent brain damage or death
    2. Interventions

CLINICAL ALERT

      a. Meet basic physiologic needs
      b. Keep the patient safe
        (1) Never leave a disoriented patient alone
        (2) Make sure someone is always with him to prevent injury
      c. Institute measures to help patient relax and fall asleep
      d. Keep room lit
      e. Protect patient from self-harm
      f. Reorient patient; explain that he is sick and in the hospital
      g. Determine family's perception of events and clarify any misconceptions or inaccuracies

E. Evaluation
    1. Base the evaluation on an accurate identification of the problem
    2. Determine if individual goals have been developed and achieved

◆ II. Dementia

A. Description
    1. Dementia is a global impairment of cognitive functioning, memory, and personality without disturbance in level of consciousness caused by irreversible alteration in brain function
    2. There are more than 70 different kinds of dementia, including ALZHEIMER'S disease, Pick's disease, Huntington's disease, acquired immunodeficiency syndrome, Korsakoff's disease, and Parkinson's disease
    3. The onset of dementia is gradual with slow, continuous decline; dementia ends in death
    4. Behaviors seen reflect brain tissue alteration

    5. Alzheimer's disease accounts for 50% of dementia in old age

    6. Usually, families are the primary caregivers

B. Nursing assessment

  1. Behavioral characteristics

    a. Stage I

      (1) Decline in recent memory

      (2) Agitated or apathetic

      (3) Wanders

      (4) Decline in personal appearance

      (5) Frightened

      (6) Attempts to cover up symptoms

    b. Stage II

      (1) Socially unacceptable behavior

      (2) Poor impulse control

      (3) Tantrums

      (4) Becomes lost when wandering

      (5) Requires assistance with activities of daily living

      (6) Increased appetite with no weight gain

      (7) Continuous, repetitive behaviors

    c. Stage III

      (1) HYPERORALITY

      (2) BULIMIA NERVOSA

      (3) Compulsive touching and examination of objects

      (4) Deterioration in motor ability

  2. Affective characteristics

    a. Stage I

      (1) Anxiety

      (2) Depression

      (3) Helplessness

      (4) Frustration

      (5) Shame

      (6) Lack of spontaneous communication

    b. Stage II

      (1) Emotional lability

      (2) Fear

      (3) Catastrophic reactions

    c. Stage III

      (1) Decreased response to stimuli

      (2) Nonresponsive

  3. Cognitive characteristics

    a. Stage I

      (1) Impaired memory

      (2) Decreased concentration

      (3) Easily distracted

        (4) Absentminded

        (5) Decreased ability to make accurate judgments

        (6) Disoriented regarding time

        (7) Transitory delusions of persecution

     b. Stage II

        (1) Has progressive memory loss

        (2) Is unable to retain new information

        (3) Does not recognize family members

        (4) Exhibits CONFABULATION

        (5) Has diminished comprehension

        (6) Is disoriented X 3

        (7) Has increased loss of ability to understand or use language

     c. Stage III

        (1) Experiences severe decline in cognitive functioning

        (2) Is unable to speak

        (3) Lacks nonverbal response to stimuli

        (4) Enters vegetative stage

  4. Physiologic characteristics

     a. Stage I

        (1) Muscular twitching

        (2) Loss of energy

        (3) Fatigue

        (4) Disturbed sleep

        (5) Susceptible to falls

     b. Stage II

        (1) Incontinence of bowel and bladder

        (2) Decreased reaction time

     c. Stage III

        (1) Emaciation

        (2) Death

C. Diagnoses

  1. Related *DSM-IV* medical diagnoses

     a. Dementia of the Alzheimer's type

     b. Vascular dementia

     c. Substance-induced persisting dementia

     d. Dementia due to multiple etiologies

  2. Primary NANDA nursing diagnosis: Altered thought process

D. Nursing planning and implementation

  1. Outcomes

     a. Patient will achieve optimum level of cognitive functioning

     b. Patient will remain free from harm

  2. Interventions

     a. Increase social interaction

TEACHING TIPS
Patient with Alzheimer's disease

Be sure to include the following topics in your teaching plan for the patient with Alzheimer's disease and his family.
- Definition of dementia
- Definition of the spheres of orientation
- Symptoms and usual course of Alzheimer's disease
- Medications
- Dealing with disorientation, impaired communication, aggressive behavior, loss of self-care abilities
- Safety in the home
- Stress reduction for caregivers
- Use of community resources

    b. Promote physical activity
    c. Provide sensory stimulation
    d. Reorient to reality
    e. Use a night light
    f. Talk about remote memories

CLINICAL ALERT

    g. Use clear, concise, unhurried verbal communication
    h. Provide verbal and nonverbal communication that is congruent; consistency and structure are crucial to prevent added confusion and to maintain patient safety
    i. Encourage reminiscence
    j. Provide a structured environment
    k. State expectations simply and completely
    l. Offer support and education to caregivers (See *Patient with Alzheimer's disease*)
    m. Encourage use of community resources; make appropriate referrals as necessary

  E. Evaluation
    1. Base evaluation on goals and achievements; update goals as behaviors change
    2. Determine alternative approaches used

POINTS TO REMEMBER

◆ Delirium occurs in all ages, but incidence increases with advanced age.

◆ Nursing assessment must include family's perceptions with delirium.

◆ Measures must be taken to prevent permanent brain damage or death.

◆ Families are usually the primary caregivers for people with dementia.

◆ Keeping the patient with cognitive impairment safe is a priority.

STUDY QUESTIONS

To evaluate your understanding of this chapter, answer the following questions in the space provided; then compare your responses with the correct answers in Appendix B pages 174 and 175.

1. What are four behavioral characteristics of delirium? _____

   _____

   _____

2. What is the primary NANDA diagnosis for patients with cognitive impairment disorders? _____

   _____

   _____

3. What is the primary nursing care goal for a patient with delirium? _____

   _____

   _____

4. Which is the most common kind of dementia seen in older people?_____

   _____

   _____

5. What are four nursing interventions for patients with dementia? _____

   _____

   _____

CRITICAL THINKING AND APPLICATION EXERCISES

1. Develop a table comparing delirium and dementia.

2. Interview a family caring for a patient with Alzheimer's disease. Prepare an oral presentation describing the family's typical day.

3. Develop a plan of care from admission through discharge for a patient with a cognitive impairment disorder. Be sure to include plans for education and follow-up.

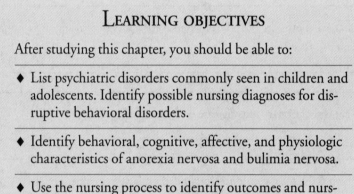

Childhood and Adolescent Disorders

LEARNING OBJECTIVES

After studying this chapter, you should be able to:

♦ List psychiatric disorders commonly seen in children and adolescents. Identify possible nursing diagnoses for disruptive behavioral disorders.

♦ Identify behavioral, cognitive, affective, and physiologic characteristics of anorexia nervosa and bulimia nervosa.

♦ Use the nursing process to identify outcomes and nursing interventions for selected psychiatric disorders commonly seen in children and adolescents.

CHAPTER OVERVIEW

Psychiatric disorders in children and adolescents seriously interfere with personal, family, and social adjustments. Accurate and thorough assessment is necessary to differentiate between normal and abnormal behavior. Nursing outcomes and interventions must be individual and must consider the developmental level of the patient. Parents with children experiencing psychiatric disorders require support and education from professional and community sources.

♦ I. Mental retardation

A. Description
1. Significant subaverage intelligence categorized by IQ below 70
   a. Mild = IQ 55 to 69
   b. Moderate = IQ 40 to 54
   c. Severe = IQ 25 to 39
   d. Profound = IQ below 24
2. Etiology unclear
3. Secondary psychopathology often evident

B. Nursing assessment
1. Ability to meet developmental milestones
2. Results of psychological and educational testing
3. Ability to verbalize and relate to others
4. Ability to verbalize needs and express emotions
5. Ability to solve problems
6. Ability to care for self
7. Degree of acting-out behaviors

C. Diagnoses
1. Related *DSM-IV* medical diagnoses
   a. Mild mental retardation
   b. Moderate mental retardation
   c. Severe mental retardation
   d. Profound mental retardation
   e. Unspecified severity of mental retardation
2. Related NANDA nursing diagnoses
   a. Altered growth and development
   b. Impaired verbal communication
   c. Impaired social interaction
   d. Altered family processes
   e. Self-care deficit
   f. Self-esteem disturbance

D. Nursing planning and implementation
1. Outcomes
   a. Patient will achieve maximum level of functioning possible
   b. Patient and family will confirm use of community services
   c. Family will demonstrate positive coping mechanisms
   d. Patient will demonstrate a decrease in socially unacceptable or destructive behaviors

2. Nursing interventions
   a. Implement various interventions depending on patient's level of retardation and additional psychopathology
   b. Assist with referrals to community resources for screening and assessment
   c. Provide emotional support for parents
   d. Encourage use of community services
   e. Assist with behavior modification
   f. Provide psychoeducation for family
   g. Assist with treatment modalities as appropriate
      (1) Recommend crisis interaction for family
      (2) Teach stress management
      (3) Recommend parenting groups

E. Evaluation
   1. Perform an early and accurate assessment
   2. Determine the level of family education and support
   3. Determine the family's use of community resources
   4. Measure the patient's decrease in socially unacceptable or destructive behaviors

♦ II. Autistic disorder (AD)

A. Description
   1. AD is a pervasive developmental disorder
   2. The disorder is a severe impairment of social interactions and imaginative activities
   3. The disorder becomes obvious between 18 to 36 months of age
   4. Majority of those with the disorder have an IQ between 35 to 50

B. Nursing assessment
   1. Little to no communication with others
   2. Ritualistic behavior
   3. Repetitive behavior
   4. Disturbed motor behavior (rocking, whirling)
   5. Stereotypic behavior (finger snapping)
   6. Head banging
   7. Unpredictable moods

C. Diagnoses
   1. Related *DSM-IV* medical diagnoses
      a. Pervasive developmental disorder
      b. Autistic disorder
   2. Related NANDA nursing diagnoses
      a. Altered family processes
      b. Impaired social interaction

    c. Impaired physical mobility
    d. Risk for violence: self-directed

D. Nursing planning and implementation
  1. Outcomes
    a. Child will exhibit modification in coping responses
    b. Child will demonstrate strengthening of competency skills
    c. Family will demonstrate use of appropriate communication skills
  2. Interventions
    a. Establish trusting relationship
    b. Assign a team of staff to develop consistency
    c. Provide age appropriate play therapy
    d. Be attentive without being intrusive
    e. Talk face to face with child so that the child focuses on the conversation and is not distracted
    f. Attempt to establish a relationship between the child and family, and teach effective communication skills

CLINICAL ALERT

E. Evaluation
  1. Evaluation of child may be difficult because of communication problems
  2. Determine if there is a decrease in repetitive, ritualistic behavior

♦ III. General disruptive behavior disorders

A. Description
  1. Socially disruptive and inappropriate behavior
  2. Behaviors related to inattention
  3. Behaviors inconsistent with developmental level

B. Types
  1. Attention deficit hyperactivity disorder (ADHD)
    a. Description
      (1) Inattention
      (2) Short attention span
      (3) Distractibility
      (4) Learning disabilities (common)
      (5) Possible hallucinations
    b. Nursing assessment
      (1) Infants
        (a) Difficulty sleeping
        (b) Active in the crib
        (c) Frequent crying
        (d) Rapid development
        (e) Rapid, impulsive activity

(2) Toddlers
   (a) Unable to sit still
   (b) Trail of destruction
   (c) Unable to stop activity (will not sit down to eat)
(3) Children
   (a) Labile mood
   (b) Explosive irritability
   (c) Negative self-concept
   (d) Difficulty forming relationships
2. Attention deficit without hyperactivity disorder
   a. Description
      (1) No hyperactivity
      (2) Primarily cognitive symptoms
         (a) Inattention
         (b) Short attention span
         (c) Distractibility
         (d) Possible learning disabilities
   b. Nursing assessment
      (1) Inattention
      (2) Distractibility
3. CONDUCT DISORDER
   a. Description
      (1) Severe, persistent antisocial behavior
      (2) Lack of guilt or remorse
      (3) Social alienation
      (4) Lack of social controls
   b. Nursing assessment
      (1) Often physically aggressive
      (2) May exhibit cruelty to others and animals
      (3) Often in trouble with authority
      (4) Outward-directed anger
      (5) Truancy
      (6) Manipulativeness
4. Oppositional defiant disorder
   a. Description
      (1) Disruptive behavior occurring more frequently and lasting longer than usual behavioral problems of peers
      (2) Social problems with peers and adults
      (3) Possibly a milder form of conduct disorder
   b. Nursing assessment
      (1) Disruptive and argumentative
      (2) Hostile and irritable
      (3) Defying rules
      (4) Blaming problems on others

        (5) Impaired academic functioning
        (6) Seeking instant gratification

C. Diagnoses
  1. Related *DSM-IV* medical diagnoses
    a. Attention deficit hyperactivity disorder
      (1) Predominantly inattentive type
      (2) Predominantly hyperactive-impulsive type
      (3) Combined type
      (4) Not otherwise specified (NOS)
    b. Opposition defiant disorder
    c. Conduct disorder
    d. Disruptive behavior disorder NOS
  2. Related NANDA nursing diagnoses
    a. Impaired social interactions
    b. Risk for violence: directed at others
    c. Altered family processes
    d. Altered thought processes
    e. Self-esteem disturbance
    f. Social isolation

D. Nursing planning and implementation
  1. Outcomes
    a. Patient will demonstrate measures to delay gratification
    b. Patient will exhibit improved social interaction skills
    c. Patient will demonstrate more appropriate coping skills

**INICAL
ALERT**

  2. Nursing interventions
    a. Assist with behavior management strategies
    b. Use stories and play to assist in coping with frustration
    c. Use MODELING to elicit cooperative behavior
    d. Reinforce cooperative behavior
    e. Do not humiliate or use shame; doing so is intimidating and would serve only to demean and lower the child's self-esteem
    f. State expectations
    g. Encourage verbal expression of needs and goals
    h. Avoid judgmental statements
    i. Set limits; discuss and implement appropriate consequences
    j. Expect reciprocal respect

E. Evaluation
  1. Determine if patient has increased coping skills
  2. Determine if patient has decreased disruptive behavior
  3. Measure for more appropriate social interaction skills
  4. Check for improved school performance

♦ IV. Anxiety disorders

A. Description
  1. Rare in childhood
  2. Usually short-lived disorders
  3. A disorder when normal development is disrupted

B. Types
  1. Separation anxiety disorder
    a. Description
      (1) Common in a mild form
      (2) Develops at any age
      (3) More commonly seen in children
    b. Nursing assessment
      (1) Needs to be physically near parent
      (2) Worries about being kidnapped or killed, or parent being killed
      (3) Refuses to go to school
      (4) Has physiologic symptoms including nausea, vomiting, stomachache, sore throat, respiratory distress, dizziness
  2. School phobia disorder
    a. Description
      (1) Is more common in girls
      (2) Is characterized by excessive fear of unfamiliar people and situations
      (3) May extend into adolescence and early adulthood
    b. Nursing assessment
      (1) Shy
      (2) Hides from or refuses to speak to strangers
      (3) Whispers
      (4) Blushes easily
      (5) Avoids competition
  3. Generalized anxiety disorder
    a. Description
      (1) Is more common in girls
      (2) Is characterized by intense need to succeed
    b. Nursing assessment
      (1) Expresses excessive worry
      (2) Expresses unrealistic concerns over past and future events
      (3) Exhibits perfectionism
      (4) Seeks frequent reassurance
      (5) Engages in nail biting, hair pulling, foot tapping

4. Obsessive-compulsive disorder
   a. Description
      (1) Symptoms are similar to those seen in adults
      (2) Child is not able to recognize connection between obsessive thoughts and compulsive behavior
   b. Nursing assessment
      (1) Has obsessive thoughts
      (2) Engages in compulsive behaviors (i.e. repeatedly redoes homework, spends excessive amount of time on activities of daily living)
      (3) Tries to hide symptoms

C. Diagnoses
   1. Related *DSM-IV* medical diagnoses
      a. Separation anxiety disorder
      b. Reactive attachment disorder of infancy or early childhood
      c. Generalized anxiety disorder
      d. Obsessive-compulsive disorder
   2. Related NANDA nursing diagnoses
      a. Anxiety
      b. Fear
      c. Chronic low self-esteem
      d. Ineffective individual coping

D. Nursing planning and implementation
   1. Outcomes
      a. Patient will demonstrate modified coping responses
      b. Patient will exhibit strengthened competency skills
   2. Nursing interventions
      a. Offer frequent exercise
      b. Encourage decision making
      c. Help child identify fears by using art, books, and play
      d. Reinforce social interaction
      e. Redirect behavior to restore self-control

E. Evaluation
   1. Development of new coping skills
   2. Decrease in anxiety

◆ V. Eating disorders

A. Description
   1. Predisposing factors include distorted body image with fear of becoming fat, low self-esteem, and preoccupation with weight and dieting
   2. ANOREXIA NERVOSA is an eating disorder characterized by deliberate starvation to become as thin as possible

3. BULIMIA NERVOSA is an eating disorder characterized by episodic binging and then purging
4. An individual can have both anorexia nervosa and bulimia nervosa
5. Of the people experiencing eating disorders, 90% to 95% are female
6. Eating disorders usually develop during adolescence

B. Types
  1. Anorexia nervosa
    a. Description
      (1) Disorder is characterized by severe underweight
      (2) Persons with anorexia nervosa are attempting to control themselves and their environment
      (3) Person dramatically decreases food intake
      (4) Person sharply increases physical exercise
      (5) Disorder may end in death
    b. Nursing assessment
      (1) Behavioral characteristics
        (a) Needs to please others
        (b) Is overly compliant
        (c) Is an overachiever
        (d) Has obsessive ritual
        (e) Refuses to eat
        (f) Has phobias
        (g) Exhibits compulsive behavior
        (h) Is a perfectionist
        (i) Has rigid rules
      (2) Affective characteristics
        (a) Is fearful
        (b) Feels guilty when eating
        (c) Depends on others for self-worth
      (3) Cognitive characteristics
        (a) Has cognitive distortions, such as selective abstraction, overgeneralization, magnification, ideas of reference, dichotomous thinking, distorted body image, and ALEXITHYMIA
        (b) Exhibits self-depreciation
        (c) Shows impaired decision making
      (4) Physiologic characteristics
        (a) Electrolyte imbalance evidenced by muscle weakness, seizures, arrhythmias
        (b) Decreased blood volume evidenced by lowered blood pressure, postural hypertension
        (c) G.I. complications including constipation, cathartic color, laxative dependence

    (d) Amenorrhea
    (e) Weight loss
2. Bulimia nervosa
  a. Description
    (1) Weight is normal or near-normal
    (2) Binge eating cycles are followed by purging
    (3) Severity of disorder depends on frequency of cycle
    (4) Develops around ages 17 to 23
    (5) Food is used as a source of comfort
  b. Nursing assessment
    (1) Behavioral characteristics
      (a) Focuses on changing specific body part
      (b) Binges
      (c) PURGES
      (d) Engages in overly strict dieting
      (e) May use amphetamines and street drugs to control hunger
      (f) Sporadically exercises excessively
      (g) May steal to get money to buy food
      (h) Relationships are disrupted
      (i) Often lies and makes excuses
    (2) Affective characteristics
      (a) Needs acceptance and approval
      (b) Represses anger and frustration
      (c) Avoids conflict
      (d) Is fearful
      (e) Is anxious
      (f) Exhibits guilt and self-disgust
    (3) Cognitive characteristics
      (a) Is troubled by own behavior
      (b) Feels helpless to stop
      (c) Is always thinking about food
      (d) Shows the same cognitive distortions as seen in anorexia nervosa
      (e) Is a perfectionist
    (4) Physiologic characteristics
      (a) Similar to those seen in anorexia nervosa
      (b) Problems from frequent vomiting, such as esophagitis, possible gastric rupture, dental caries, tooth loss, chronic sore throat, swollen salivary glands
      (c) Irregular menses
C. Diagnoses
  1. Related *DSM-IV* medical diagnoses
    a. Anorexia nervosa
    b. Bulimia nervosa

TEACHING TIPS
Patient with an eating disorder

Be sure to include the following topics in your teaching plan for the patient with an eating disorder.
• Underlying issues surrounding the eating disorder
• Possible long-term complications
• Need for gradual weight gain
• Nutritional support measures
• Treatment options
• Support services and community resources

    c. Eating disorder NOS
  2. Related NANDA nursing diagnoses
    a. Altered nutrition: Less than body requirements
    b. Anxiety
    c. Altered thought process
    d. Disturbed body image
    e. Impaired social interaction
    f. Risk for injury
    g. Powerlessness
    h. Ineffective individual coping

D. Nursing planning and implementation
  1. Outcomes
    a. Patient will exhibit improved nutritional status
    b. Patient will demonstrate use of appropriate coping mechanisms
    c. Patient will remain physically safe
    d. Patient will develop healthy eating habits
  2. Nursing interventions

CLINICAL ALERT

    a. Obtain a complete physical assessment
    b. Contract for amount to be eaten; avoid power struggles around food because the focus is establishing and maintaining positive self-image and self-esteem
    c. Prevent patient from using bathroom for 2 hours after eating
    d. Provide one-on-one support before, during, and after meals
    e. Reassure patient that excess weight gain will not happen
    f. Encourage verbal expression of feelings

CLINICAL ALERT

    g. Help patient identify coping mechanisms for dealing with anxiety
    h. Weigh patient once or twice a week at same time of day, using the same scale
      (1) Patient should wear the same clothing to ensure accuracy of measurements.

(2) Weighing the patient too often reinforces the focus on weight rather than on the underlying issues of self-esteem.
(3) Too rapid a weight gain can be threatening to the patient.
i. Help patient identify cause of the disorder
j. Point out cognitive distortions
k. Educate patient and family (See *Patient with an eating disorder*)
E. Evaluation
1. Normalization of eating patterns
2. Development of alternate coping patterns
3. Decreased obsessive behaviors

POINTS TO REMEMBER

◆ Mental retardation is categorized as mild, moderate, severe, or profound, based on the child's IQ.

◆ Children with autistic disorders commonly exhibit little or no communication with others, disturbed motor behavior, head banging, and ritualistic, repetitive, stereotypical behavior.

◆ Attention deficit hyperactivity disorder may occur with or without hyperactivity.

◆ Anxiety becomes a disorder for a child when it disrupts normal development.

◆ The patient with bulimia nervosa uses food as a source of comfort.

STUDY QUESTIONS

To evaluate your understanding of this chapter, answer the following questions in the space provided; then compare your responses with the correct answers in Appendix B, page 175.

1. What are three nursing diagnoses for children with autistic disorder? _____
_____
_____

2. In addition to cognitive symptoms, what behaviors are commonly seen in children with attention deficit hyperactivity disorder? _____
_____
_____

3. What symptoms are most commonly seen with separation anxiety disorder? _____

_____

_____

4. What are the primary nursing outcomes for patients with eating disorders?

_____

_____

CRITICAL THINKING AND APPLICATION EXERCISES

1. Research the tools used for screening and assessing mental retardation.

2. Develop a plan for a play therapy group for children with ADHD.

3. Interview a patient with an eating disorder. Write a report detailing the patient's statements and your responses. Evaluate your interaction with the
patient.

4. Develop a plan of care from admission through discharge for a patient
with a childhood or adolescent psychiatric disorder. Be sure to include
plans for education and follow-up.

Glossary

Adaptation—organism's adjustment to its environment

Addiction—compulsive use of a chemical substance that contributes to physical or psychological dependence

Affect—outward manifestation of emotions

Aggression—mental drive that can lead to constructive or destructive activities

Alexithymia—difficulty naming and describing emotions

Alienation—withdrawal or detachment from society

Alzheimer's disease—a chronic, progressive, incurable senile dementia involving memory loss, intellectual deterioration, personality changes, and inability to perform activities of daily living

Anhedonia—unable to experience pleasure

Anorexia nervosa—eating disorder in which person experiences hunger but refuses to eat because of a distorted body image

Anticipatory guidance—information and advice given to patients for future therapeutic purposes

Attitudinal restructuring—alteration of a position taken on an issue

Autistic thinking—ideas that have private meaning to the individual

Autogenic training—therapy that attempts to establish functional harmony by using natural forces in the brain

Automatism—spontaneous repetitive behavior or action performed without conscious control

Behavior modification—method of reeducation based on Pavlovian conditioning principles

Binge eating—rapid food consumption of large quantities in a discrete time period

Biofeedback—use of electrodes and tonal pitch to reduce tension

Body image—internalized impressions and attitudes about one's physical self

Bulimia nervosa—eating disorder with binge eating followed by vomiting or dieting

Clang association—speech pattern characterized by rhyming

Cognitive therapy—treatment approach focused on changing distorted thought processes

Community mental health—treatment philosophy advocating a comprehensive range of mental health services available to all community members

Conduct disorder—a disorder characterized by behavior that violates societal norms or the rights of others

Confabulation—behavioral reaction in which the patient creates stories or invents answers to fill in memory gaps in an unconscious attempt to maintain self-esteem

Consensual validation—reinforcement of meanings and interpretations by evidence and corroboration from others

Conversion disorder—somatoform disorder characterized by psychogenic disturbances of motor or sensory activity

Coping mechanisms—techniques used to protect oneself from the effects of anxiety

Counter-conditioning—replacement of a learned response with a less disruptive one

Crisis intervention—short-term therapy intended to reestablish a level of functioning equal to or better than the precrisis level

Defense mechanisms—unconscious coping mechanisms that a person uses to prevent awareness of anxiety or to mask feelings of inadequacy or worthlessness

Degenerative dementia—irreversible deterioration of mental capacities

Delirium—a reversible organic mental disorder with acute onset characterized by cognitive impairments and a specific stressor

Delusions—false, fixed beliefs not validated by reality and firmly held despite contradictory information

Dementia—an irreversible organic mental disorder with gradual onset characterized by cognitive impairments with or without a specific stressor

Depersonalization—feelings of estrangement and separateness from oneself

Depression—psychological state characterized by dejection, lowered self-esteem, hopelessness, helplessness, indecision, and rumination

Desensitization—gradual exposure to a predetermined stress-producing stimulus on a continuum from least to most severe

Dichotomous thinking—categorization of events, objects, or ideas into two, usually opposing parts

Echolalia—purposeless repetition of a word or phrase just spoken by someone else

Ego-dystonic behaviors—behaviors that disrupt one's identity or sense of self

Ego-syntonic behaviors—behaviors that are compatible with one's identity or sense of self

Empathy—ability to understand the feelings of others and to respond sensitively

Encounter group therapy—therapy that focuses on the reaction of members to events in the group

Exhibitionism—sexual gratification obtained through public exposure of the genitals

Existentialism—school of philosophical thought that focuses on the present and presumes that a person finds meaning in life through experiences

Fear—emotional reaction to an environmental threat; feeling of dread

Feedback—process by which functioning is monitored, corrected (if inappropriate), and maintained (if appropriate)

Fight-or-flight response—sympathetic nervous system response to anxiety in which an individual deals with a stressful situation or avoids it

Free association—psychoanalytic technique in which the patient articulates all thoughts

Gestalt therapy—therapy that focuses on enhancement of self-awareness

Grieving—subjective response to the loss of a highly valued person or object

Guided imagery—therapy that controls anxiety by helping the patient visualize successful coping with a stressful event

Hallucination—occurrence of sight, sound, touch, smell, or taste without any external stimulus

Holistic—viewing a human being as a unified biologic, psychological, and social organism

Hostility—anger and resentment characterized by destructive behavior

Hydrotherapy—use of wet sheet packs or 2- to 10-hour tub baths for psychotherapeutic purposes

Hyperonality—need to taste, chew, and examine any object small enough to be placed in the mouth

Hypochondriasis—depression marked by a persistent fear or belief that one has a serious illness

Hypnosis—a treatment modality in which the patient, in a sleeplike state, experiences abnormal sensibility to the hypnotist's suggestions.

Id—mental structure in psychoanalytic theory that represents unconscious drives and impulses

Identity—sense of selfhood that sustains an integrated personality structure

Incest—sexual relationship between persons who are biologically related

Lethality—the degree to which a suicide attempt will result in death

Magical thinking—belief that one's thoughts or wishes can control other people or events

Mania—psychological state characterized by an elevated or expansive mood

Milieu—social and cultural aspects of the treatment setting that can reduce behavioral disturbances

Milieu therapy—manipulation of a patient's sociocultural environment to reduce behavioral disturbances

Modeling—technique used to help a patient develop new behaviors by observing and copying the behaviors of others

Mutism—lack of speech

Narcotherapy—induction of state of sedation by intravenous administration of sedatives or stimulants

Neologism—invented word understood only by the inventor

Neurotic behavior—dysfunctional behavior characterized by anxiety without reality distortion

Neurotransmitter—chemical substance that carries impulses between neurons

Operant conditioning—behavior modification through systematic manipulation of antecedents and consequences

Perception—response of sensory receptors to external stimuli that involves both cognitive and emotional knowledge

Phototherapy—exposure to full-spectrum fluorescent lamps for treatment of seasonal affective disorder

Primary prevention—actions taken to reduce the incidence of disease

Projection—attribution of blame or responsibility for one's acts and feelings to other people

Psychodrama—structured, directed dramatization of a patient's personal, emotional, and interactional problems

Psychogenic fugue—maladaptive response to a problem with self-concept in which the patient assumes a new identity after sudden, unexpected travel away from home or work

Psychogenic pain—pain originating in the mind

Psychological autopsy—a process by which the survivors of a suicide victim review the event and their reactions to it

Psychological dependence—subjective feeling that a certain object is necessary for well-being

Psychosis—psychological state in which the ability to recognize reality, communicate, and relate to others is seriously impaired

Psychosurgery—surgical interruption of neural pathways in the brain associated with transmission of emotional impulses

Psychotic behavior—severely dysfunctional behavior characterized by panic anxiety, personality disintegration, and regressive behavior

Purge—prevention of weight gain by behaviors such as vomiting, excessive exercise, or use of diet pills, diuretics or laxatives

Rational-emotive therapy—therapy that focuses on risk taking and on assuming responsibility for one's behavior

Reaction formation—use of behaviors that are opposite to what one would like to do

Reality therapy—therapy that focuses on recognition and accomplishment of life goals, emphasizing development of capacity to care about self and others

Relationship therapy—one-on-one nurse-patient relationship in which the nursing process is used to meet the patient's needs

Resistance—tendency to maintain maladaptive behaviors despite therapeutic intervention

Role clarification—gaining of knowledge in order to perform a specific role

Role modeling—performing a certain role in a manner that warrants emulation

Role playing—acting out a situation in order to deepen one's ability to see from another point of view

Role reversal—acting out the role of another person with whom one is in conflict

Rumination—persistent thinking about and discussion of a particular idea or subject

Schizoaffective disorder—medical diagnosis that denotes symptoms of schizophrenia coupled with an altered mood (usually depression)

Seasonal affective disorder (SAD)—a mood disorder characterized by depression during fall and winter, and normal mood or hypomania during spring and summer

Seclusion—placement of an agitated patient alone in a single room (sometimes locked) to decrease stimuli and to allow the patient time to regain control

Secondary prevention—actions taken to reduce the prevalence of disease

Selective inattention—process of tuning out details associated with anxiety-producing situations

Self-actualization—fulfilling one's potential

Self-awareness—recognition of what one experiences and how one reacts to the experiences

Self-concept—all knowledge and beliefs held about oneself in relation to one's physical and social environment

Self-destructive behavior—behavior that is intended to harm or destroy self

Self-esteem—feelings held about oneself in relation to personal worth and value

Semantic fallacies—misperceptions, distortions, and irrational beliefs that contribute to automatic negative thinking, commonly present in depressed patients

Somatic therapies—treatments that affect physiological functioning, such as psychosurgery, electroconvulsive therapy, pharmacotherapy

Somatoform disorders—disorders characterized by recurrent and multiple physical symptoms that have no organic or physiologic base

Stressors—stimuli that one perceives as challenging, threatening, or demanding; may be pleasant or unpleasant, internal or external, physiologic or psychosocial

Suicide—conscious act of self-induced annihilation

Suicide ideation—thought of self-induced annihilation

Superego—mental structure in psychoanalytic theory that evaluates actions of the ego

Supportive confrontation—technique used to make a patient aware of incongruences in attitudes, feelings, or behaviors by verbalizing observed discrepancies

Symbolization—defense mechanism in which an abstract representation is made of an actual object

Tangentiality—form of speech, common in schizophrenics, in which the response to a question begins appropriately but then deviates from the topic to related matters

Tertiary prevention—actions taken to reduce disability associated with disease

Therapeutic touch—Laying a hand on or close to the body of an ill person for the purpose of healing

Token economy system—a form of behavior modification in which an object is used as positive reinforcement to promote behavioral change

Tolerance—state characterized by the need for increasingly larger doses of a drug to obtain the effects previously obtained at lower doses

Transference—projection of feelings about significant others onto the therapist

Transmethylation—molecular transformation of one catecholamine to another

Uncomplicated grief reaction—healthy, adaptive response to loss; resolved when the lost person or object is internalized, the bonds of attachment are loosened, and new relationships are established

Undoing—use of an act or utterance to negate, at least partially, a previous act or utterance

Violence—extreme force or destructive action that injures or hurts others

Visualization—use of positive mental images to consciously program a desired change

Withdrawal syndrome—collection of symptoms that occur after cessation of an abused substance

Word salad—communication pattern characterized by a jumble of disconnected words

Answers to Study Questions

1. During the late 1800s and early 1900s, nursing care focused on providing custodial care, meeting the patient's physical needs, dispensing medications, assisting with hydrotherapy, and encouraging patient participation in ward activities.

2. The National Mental Health Act of 1946 created the NIMH.

3. During the 1960s and 1970s, treatment for mentally ill persons moved from institutions to the community.

4. The ANA defines the psychiatric nursing role as a specialized area of nursing practice that employs theories of human behavior as its science and the "powerful use of self" as its art.

5. In primary prevention, psychiatric nursing functions include health education, improvement of socioeconomic conditions, consumer education about normal growth and development, referral before symptoms develop, support of family members, and community and political activity.

6. Psychiatric nurse generalists have baccalaureate education. They meet the profession's standards of knowledge, experience, and quality of care. Specialists have graduate education, supervised clinical experience, and a depth of knowledge, competence, and skill in practice.

CHAPTER 2

1. The behavioral model is based on the concept that all behavior is learned.

2. In the existential model, the therapist and the patient are equals, with the therapist acting as a guide.

3. The six phases of interpersonal development are infancy (ages 1 to 2), childhood (ages 2 to 6), juvenile (ages 6 to 9), preadolescence (ages 9 to 12), early adolescence (ages 12 to 15), and late adolescence (ages 15 to 21).

4. The medical model uses the *Diagnostic and Statistical Manual of Mental Disorders, Fourth Edition* (*DSM-IV*) of the American Psychiatric Association to record and classify diagnoses.

5. Nursing models focus on the patient's biological, psychological, and sociocultural needs and on the nurse's caring functions.

6. Sigmund Freud is considered the father of the psychoanalytic model.

7. In the social model, the patient initiates therapy and defines the problem. The therapist collaborates with the patient to pro-

mote change, while advocating
freedom of choice and community mental health.

CHAPTER 3

1. Crisis occurs when stress overwhelms the individual's usual
coping mechanisms. It is self-
limiting, typically resolving
within 6 weeks.
2. Crisis intervention increases the
likelihood that a crisis will be
positively resolved, offers immediate help and reestablishes equilibrium, can restore the patient's
precrisis level of functioning,
and teaches the patient effective
problem-solving skills.
3. In the therapeutic environment,
the nurse acts primarily in inpatient settings to facilitate and
oversee implementation of interventions, to act as a role model,
and to structure the patient's environment.
4. Membership roles in groups include task roles, maintenance
roles, and egocentric roles.
5. The focus of family therapy is on
family interaction.
6. The clinical nurse specialist acts
as a psychotherapist during therapy; the nurse generalist acts as a
supportive therapist, counseling
the patient and maintaining the
nurse-patient relationship.
7. Biological therapies focus on
symptoms, diagnoses, and prog-
noses.

CHAPTER 4

1. Stress is a state of imbalance
within an organism brought
about by an actual or perceived

disparity between environmental
demands (called stressors) and
the organism's capacity to cope
with them.
2. The stress response is influenced
by the intensity and duration of
the stressful stimulus and by the
person's perception of control
over the stimulus.
3. The three phases of general adaptation syndrome are alarm, resistance, and exhaustion.
4. *DSM-IV* medical diagnoses and
NANDA nursing diagnoses are
used to identify stress and psy-
chobiologic disorders.
5. Stress management strategies include progressive relaxation, biofeedback, meditation, hypnosis,
guided imagery, behavior modification, yoga, exercise and stretching, attitudinal restructuring,
autogenic training, stress desensitization, massage, therapeutic
touch, psychotherapy, nutrition,
laughter, play, and music.

CHAPTER 5

1. The five stages of coping with an
anticipated death are denial, anger, bargaining, depression, and
acceptance.
2. Nursing care goals focus on helping the patient to live more fully
and comfortably until death,
supporting the family, and promoting acceptance of death.
3. The three phases of uncomplicated grief are shock and disbe-
lief; heightened awareness; and
reorganization, letting go, and
resolution.
4. Symptoms of grief that are important in evaluating a grieving pa-

tient include somatic distress, preoccupation with the deceased, guilt and hostility, and personality disorganization.

5. The nurse sets goals according to the patient's needs, then directs interventions toward specific behaviors.

CHAPTER 6

1. A person's self-concept includes body image, identity, roles, self-esteem, and self-ideals.

2. The three behavioral categories associated with an altered self-concept are low self-esteem, identity confusion, and depersonalization.

3. The primary nursing outcomes for a patient with an altered self-concept are to increase the patient's self-realization and self-acceptance while helping the patient demonstrate increased confidence and self-worth.

4. When assisting the patient with self-evaluation, the nurse should help identify relevant stressors, unrealistic goals, faulty perceptions, strengths, coping resources, and maladaptive responses. To accomplish this, the nurse can use such techniques as facilitative communication, supportive confrontation, role clarification, and psychodrama.

CHAPTER 7

1. Six affective responses to anxiety include edginess, impatience, uneasiness, tension, fear, and jumpiness.

2. When caring for a patient experiencing panic, the nurse must re-

main calm and try to reduce the patient's anxiety.

3. To be diagnosed with a generalized anxiety state, a patient must be at least age 18.

4. The key sign of phobia is panic when the patient sees the feared object.

5. Key signs and symptoms of a patient with an obsessive-compulsive disorder include repetitive thoughts that the person cannot control or exclude from consciousness; recurring, irresistible impulses to perform an action; and defense mechanisms, such as isolation, undoing, reaction formation, and magical thinking.

6. When caring for a patient with a post-traumatic stress disorder, the nurse should explore the meaning of the event, assist with problem solving, teach relaxation techniques, provide for patient safety, and encourage patient to join support groups.

7. Nursing interventions for a patient with a dissociative disorder should focus on the patient and not on the symptoms.

CHAPTER 8

1. Biological etiologies for mood disorders include biogenic amine hypothesis, electrolyte metabolism disturbance, neuroendocrine abnormalities, catecholamine imbalance, and a disturbance in biological rhythms.

2. Martin Seligman postulated the learned helplessness concept.

3. The six special treatment measures for mood disorders include electroconvulsive therapy, antide-

pressant medications, lithium therapy, group and individual therapies, phototherapy, and sleep manipulation.

4. Cognitive changes for a patient experiencing moderate depression include slow thinking and a narrowing of interests, indecisiveness, self-doubt, rumination, and pessimism.

5. The critical nursing intervention is to assess the depressed patient's suicide risk.

6. Nursing care outcomes for a manic patient include patient not harming self or others; patient monitoring own behavior and exercising self-control; and patient maintaining an adequate balance of rest, sleep, and nutrition.

CHAPTER 9

1. High-risk factors include being an adolescent, male, elderly, or substance abuser; having rejected treatment or being noncompliant with treatment; being depressed or schizophrenic; having a terminal or chronic illness; having psychological stresses or certain personality traits; having made previous suicide attempts.

2. Three categories of pharmacologic agents used to treat suicidal patients are antidepressants, antianxiety agents, and antimanic agents.

3. The nurse would determine the appropriate level of suicide precautions and explain them to the patient; assess suicide potential daily; re-evaluate the level of precautions daily; obtain assessment data in a matter-of-fact manner; ask the patient directly about the suicide plan; remove dangerous objects from the area; place the patient in a room near the nurses' station, in view of staff; make sure windows are locked; and stay close to the patient when sharp objects must be used.

4. Family nursing care interventions include lessening the long-term effects of grieving and promoting grieving; recognizing that support from friends may be lacking; helping the family explore their guilt; being alert to "anniversary suicide" by relatives; and helping the family deal with hostility and destructiveness.

CHAPTER 10

1. Psychotic behavior includes various symptoms resulting from disturbed thought process, distorted perceptions, brain damage, or chemical toxicity.

2. The sequential steps of schizophrenia are inability to trust, dissociation, displacement, fantasy, and projection.

3. Primary manifestations of schizophrenia include associative looseness, autistic thinking, ambivalence, and alterations of affect.

4. Hallucinations develop in three phases: the patient focuses on comforting thoughts to relieve anxiety and stress; experiences outward projection; and experiences increasing preoccupation and helplessness. The hallucination is controlling but comfort-

ing, although content may become menacing.

5. Behavioral manifestations of schizophrenia include withdrawal, regression, overactivity or underactivity, impulsivity, mannerisms, automatism, and stereotypy.

6. The priority problem with a patient in an acute psychotic episode relates to basic physical and safety needs.

7. Principles of therapeutic interaction include acceptance of the patient, acknowledgment, authenticity, and self-awareness.

8. To help the patient establish ego boundaries, the nurse would validate a patient's real perceptions and correct misconceptions matter-of-factly; avoid arguing; stay with a frightened patient; discuss simple, concrete topics; and provide activities that help the patient maintain contact with reality.

CHAPTER 11

1. Characteristics of healthy interpersonal relationships include intimacy while maintaining separate identities; sensitivity to others' needs; mutual validation of personal worth; open communication of feelings; acceptance of others as valued, separate people; deep, empathic understanding; willingness and ability to subordinate individual needs to the needs of others or to the demands of the relationship; interdependency; and ego-syntony.

2. The young adult forms interdependent relationships, makes in-

dependent decisions, implements occupational plans, balances dependent and independent behaviors, and shows increased sensitivity to the feelings and needs of others.

3. Interventions for dependency and helplessness include anticipating the patient's needs before they demand attention; setting realistic limits; helping the patient manage anxiety; teaching the patient to express ideas and feelings assertively; supporting the patient in accepting increased decision making; and clarifying roles.

4. The key characteristic of a patient experiencing suspiciousness is an inability to trust.

5. Treatment modalities for a patient with a personality disorder may include antianxiety medications, behavior modification, and individual psychotherapy.

CHAPTER 12

1. Behavioral patterns of a substance abuser include dysfunctional anger, manipulation, impulsiveness, avoidance, and grandiosity.

2. Predisposing psychological factors of substance abuse include a dependent personality, low self-esteem, anger and frustration, feelings of omnipotence, depression, and defense mechanisms.

3. In the pre-alcoholic phase, the person uses alcohol to relax and begins to build a tolerance. In the early alcoholic phase, the person sneaks drinks, denies drinking, has feelings of guilt and in-

creasing dependency on alcohol, and blacks out. In the crucial phase, the person loses control over drinking, displays aggressive behavior, blames others for altered relationships, and has withdrawal symptoms. There also may be a loss of other interests, early morning drinking, and decreased tolerance. In the chronic phase, the person indulges in unplanned sprees; engages in solitary drinking; suffers from physical complications and impaired thinking; has no more alibis; and admits defeat. In the rehabilitative phase, the person desires help, learns alcoholism is an illness, stops drinking, begins healthy thinking, develops support systems and identifies hope for recovery. During recovery, the person develops new interests and friends, is content with sobriety, and experiences normal sleep and rest patterns and increased emotional control.

4. During withdrawal, the nurse should monitor vital signs and observe for signs of seizures and impending withdrawal syndrome.

5. Problems during the rehabilitative stage of alcoholism include denial of the illness, failure to understand the disease, low self-esteem, loneliness, low tolerance for frustration, and the possibility of relapse.

6. Behaviors associated with inhalant abuse include euphoria, decreased inhibition, misperceptions or illusions, clouding of thought, drowsiness, and rapidly

developed tolerance. No withdrawal symptoms appear.

7. Problems during an acute drug reaction include decreased circulatory and respiratory function, signs of impending withdrawal, potential for self-injury, panic and flashback reactions, and poor nutritional status.

8. The nurse can intervene during denial by focusing on the problem, avoiding the patient's attempts to focus on external problems, identifying projection of blame or defensiveness, and avoiding discussion of unanswerable questions.

CHAPTER 13

1. Functional anger energizes behavior to avoid anxiety, characterizes a healthy relationship, can project a positive self-concept, serves as an ego defense, gives a sense of control, provides immediate relief, and can indicate the need for more effective coping behaviors. Dysfunctional anger arises when early conflicts are reenacted and become a source of tension; it is cyclical and stems from or results in unresolved anger and anxiety, offensive behaviors, powerlessness, and angry responses or rejection by others.

2. Possible outcomes for a patient experiencing anger include the patient's ability to demonstrate a hierarchy of behaviors, exhibit mastery and self control, and express feelings of anger appropriately.

3. Violence carries a physical, emotional, or moral force; arouses fear in others; creates anxiety in victims; and poses a threat to safety. It may be displayed deliberately or may follow a loss of control over aggressive impulses.

4. Characteristics of a violent family system include closed boundaries; a painful and desperate mood; competition for affection, attention, and nurturance; inability of members to define themselves as individuals apart from the family system; an inability to trust; conflict within the family system; a lack of impulse control and self-discipline; a reduced capacity to delay gratification; inadequate task performance; mixed or double message communication; imbalanced power ratio; and role stereotyping.

5. Behavioral cues for child abuse include wariness of adults, rapid adaptation to the hospital unit, unwillingness to turn to parents for support, abnormal eating or drinking habits, excessive crying or none at all, and extreme fear of or total lack of respect for authority figures.

6. Motivations for sexual assault include an act of aggression; a means of gaining control; and a desire to humiliate, defile, or dominate the victim.

7. After collecting evidence in a sexual assault case, the nurse should label it carefully in the presence of a witness.

8. When intervening with a physically aggressive patient, the nurse should take precautions for personal safety and not handle the patient alone; approach the patient calmly and firmly; use short, concise statements; inform the patient what is expected; provide medication; arrange for the seclusion of the patient.

CHAPTER 14

1. Behavioral characteristics of delirium include poor impulse control; altered psychomotor activity; limited and dull, or loud and pressured speech; picking at linen and bedclothes; inability to complete tasks; bizarre, destructive behavior that worsens at night.

2. The primary NANDA nursing diagnosis for cognitive impairment disorders is altered thought process.

3. The primary nursing care goal for delirium is preventing permanent brain damage or death.

4. The most common type of dementia seen in older adults is Alzheimer's disease.

5. Nursing interventions for dementia include increasing social interaction; promoting physical activity; providing sensory stimulation; reorienting patient to reality; talking with patient about remote memories; using clear, concise, unhurried verbal communication; providing a night light; using congruent verbal and nonverbal communication; encouraging reminiscence; providing a structured environment; stating expectations sim-

ply and completely; offering support and education to caregivers; encouraging use of community resources; and making appropriate referrals.

CHAPTER 15

1. NANDA diagnoses for children with autistic disorder include altered family process; risk for self-directed violence; impaired social interaction; and impaired physical mobility.
2. Most common behaviors seen in children with attention-deficit hyperactive disorder are labile mood, explosive irritability, negative self-concept, and difficulty forming relationships.
3. There are common symptoms of separation anxiety disorder: child needs to be physically near parents; worries about being kidnapped or killed, or parent being killed; refuses to go to school; and has physiological symptoms including nausea, vomiting, stomachache, sore throat, respiratory distress, and dizziness.
4. Primary nursing outcomes for patient with eating disorders include patient's exhibiting improved nutritional status, demonstrating use of appropriate coping mechanisms, remaining physically safe, and developing healthy eating habits.

NANDA Taxonomy

The taxonomy developed by the North American Nursing Diagnosis Association (NANDA) is the currently accepted classification system for nursing diagnoses. The list of approved nursing diagnoses is grouped into nine human response patterns. The complete taxonomy is listed below.

PATTERN 1: EXCHANGING

1.1.2.1	Altered nutrition: More than body requirements
1.1.2.2	Altered nutrition: Less than body requirements
1.1.2.3	Altered nutrition: Potential for more than body requirements
1.2.1.1	Risk for infection
1.2.2.1	Risk for altered body temperature
1.2.2.2	Hypothermia
1.2.2.3	Hyperthermia
1.2.2.4	Ineffective thermo-regulation
1.2.3.1	Dysreflexia
1.3.1.1	Constipation
1.3.1.1.1	Perceived constipation
1.3.1.1.2	Colonic constipation
1.3.1.2	Diarrhea
1.3.1.3	Bowel incontinence
1.3.2	Altered urinary elimination
1.3.2.1.1	Stress incontinence
1.3.2.1.2	Reflex incontinence
1.3.2.1.3	Urge incontinence
1.3.2.1.4	Functional incontinence
1.3.2.1.5	Total incontinence
1.3.2.2	Urinary retention
1.4.1.1	Altered (specify type) tissue perfusion (renal, cerebral, cardiopulmonary, gastrointestinal, peripheral)
1.4.1.2.1	Fluid volume excess
1.4.1.2.2.1	Fluid volume deficit
1.4.1.2.2.2	Risk for fluid volume deficit
1.4.2.1	Decreased cardiac output
1.5.1.1	Impaired gas exchange
1.5.1.2	Ineffective airway clearance
1.5.1.3	Ineffective breathing pattern
1.5.1.3.1	Inability to sustain spontaneous ventilation
1.5.1.3.2	Dysfunctional ventilatory weaning response
1.6.1	Risk for injury
1.6.1.1	Risk for suffocation
1.6.1.2	Risk for poisoning
1.6.1.3	Risk for trauma
1.6.1.4	Risk for aspiration
1.6.1.5	Risk for disuse syndrome
1.6.2	Altered protection
1.6.2.1	Impaired tissue integrity
1.6.2.1.1	Altered oral mucous membrane
1.6.2.1.2.1	Impaired skin integrity
1.6.2.1.2.2	Risk for impaired skin integrity
1.7.1	Decreased adaptive capacity: Intracranial*
1.8	Energy field disturbance*

PATTERN 2: COMMUNICATING

2.1.1.1	Impaired verbal communication

*Indicates 1 of the 19 new diagnoses recently approved by NANDA.

PATTERN 3: RELATING

3.1.1	Impaired social interaction
3.1.2	Social isolation
3.1.3	Risk for loneliness*
3.2.1	Altered role performance
3.2.1.1.1	Altered parenting
3.2.1.1.2	Risk for altered parenting
3.2.1.1.2.1	Risk for altered parent/infant/child attachment*
3.2.1.2.1	Sexual dysfunction
3.2.2	Altered family processes
3.2.2.1	Caregiver role strain
3.2.2.2	Risk for caregiver role strain
3.2.2.3.1	Altered family process: Alcoholism*
3.2.3.1	Parental role conflict
3.3	Altered sexuality patterns

PATTERN 4: VALUING

4.1.1	Spiritual distress (distress of the human spirit)
4.2	Potential for enhanced spiritual well-being*

PATTERN 5: CHOOSING

5.1.1.1	Ineffective individual coping
5.1.1.1.1	Impaired adjustment
5.1.1.1.2	Defensive coping
5.1.1.1.3	Ineffective denial
5.1.2.1.1	Ineffective family coping: Disabling
5.1.2.1.2	Ineffective family coping: Compromised
5.1.2.2	Family coping: Potential for growth
5.1.3.1	Potential for enhanced community coping*
5.1.3.2	Ineffective community coping*
5.2.1	Ineffective management of therapeutic regimen: Individual
5.2.1.1	Noncompliance (specify)
5.2.2	Ineffective management of therapeutic regimen: Families*
5.2.3	Ineffective management of therapeutic regimen: Community*
5.2.4	Effective management of therapeutic regimen: Individual*
5.3.1.1	Decisional conflict (specify)
5.4	Health-seeking behaviors (specify)

PATTERN 6: MOVING

6.1.1.1	Impaired physical mobility
6.1.1.1.1	Risk for peripheral neurovascular dysfunction
6.1.1.1.2	Risk for perioperative positioning injury*
6.1.1.2	Activity intolerance
6.1.1.2.1	Fatigue
6.1.1.3	Risk for activity intolerance
6.2.1	Sleep pattern disturbance
6.3.1.1	Diversional activity deficit
6.4.1.1	Impaired home maintenance management
6.4.2	Altered health maintenance
6.5.1	Feeding self-care deficit
6.5.1.1	Impaired swallowing
6.5.1.2	Ineffective breast-feeding
6.5.1.2.1	Interrupted breast-feeding
6.5.1.3	Effective breast-feeding
6.5.1.4	Ineffective infant feeding pattern
6.5.2	Bathing or hygiene self-care deficit

*Indicates 1 of the 19 new diagnoses recently approved by NANDA.

6.5.3	Dressing or grooming self-care deficit
6.5.4	Toileting self-care deficit
6.6	Altered growth and development
6.7	Relocation stress syndrome
6.8.1	Risk for disorganized infant behavior*
6.8.2	Disorganized infant behavior*
6.8.3	Potential for enhanced organized infant behavior*

PATTERN 7: PERCEIVING

7.1.1	Body image disturbance
7.1.2	Self-esteem disturbance
7.1.2.1	Chronic low self-esteem
7.1.2.2	Situational low self-esteem
7.1.3	Personal identity disturbance
7.2	Sensory or perceptual alterations (specify visual, auditory, kinesthetic, gustatory, tactile, or olfactory)
7.2.1.1	Unilateral neglect
7.3.1	Hopelessness
7.3.2	Powerlessness

PATTERN 8: KNOWING

8.1.1	Knowledge deficit (specify)
8.2.1	Impaired environmental interpretation syndrome*
8.2.2	Acute confusion*
8.2.3	Chronic confusion*
8.3	Altered thought processes
8.3.1	Impaired memory*

PATTERN 9: FEELING

9.1.1	Pain
9.1.1.1	Chronic pain
9.2.1.1	Dysfunctional grieving
9.2.1.2	Anticipatory grieving
9.2.2	Risk for violence: Self-directed or directed at others
9.2.2.1	Risk for self-mutilation
9.2.3	Posttrauma response
9.2.3.1	Rape-trauma syndrome
9.2.3.1.1	Rape-trauma syndrome: Compound reaction
9.2.3.1.2	Rape-trauma syndrome: Silent reaction
9.3.1	Anxiety
9.3.2	Fear

*Indicates 1 of the 19 new diagnoses recently approved by NANDA.

DSM-IV
Classification

NOS = Not Otherwise Specified
An x appearing in a diagnostic code indicates that a specific code number is required.
An ellipsis (...) is used in the names of certain disorders to indicate that the name of a specific mental disorder or general medical condition should be inserted when recording the name (for example, 293.0 Delirium Due to Hypothyroidism).
If criteria are currently met, one of the following severity specifiers may be noted after the diagnosis:
– Mild
– Moderate
– Severe.
If criteria are no longer met, one of the following specifiers may be noted:
– In Partial Remission
– In Full Remission
– Prior History.

DISORDERS USUALLY FIRST DIAGNOSED IN INFANCY, CHILDHOOD, OR ADOLESCENCE

Mental Retardation
Note: These are coded on Axis II.
317   Mild Mental Retardation
318.0   Moderate Mental Retardation
318.1   Severe Mental Retardation
318.2   Profound Mental Retardation
319   Mental Retardation, Severity Unspecified

Learning Disorders
315.00 Reading Disorder
315.1   Mathematics Disorder
315.2   Disorder of Written Expression
315.9   Learning Disorder NOS

Motor Skills Disorder
315.4   Developmental Coordination Disorder

Communication Disorders
315.31 Expressive Language Disorder
315.31 Mixed Receptive-Expressive Language Disorder
315.39 Phonological Disorder
307.0   Stuttering
307.9   Communication Disorder NOS

Pervasive Developmental Disorders
299.00 Autistic Disorder
299.80 Rett's Disorder
299.10 Childhood Disintegrative Disorder
299.80 Asperger's Disorder
299.80 Pervasive Developmental Disorder NOS

Attention-Deficit and Disruptive Behavior Disorders
314.xx Attention-Deficit/ Hyperactivity Disorder
.01   Combined Type
.00   Predominantly Inattentive Type
.01   Predominantly Hyperactive-Impulsive Type

314.9 Attention-Deficit/
       Hyperactivity Disorder NOS
312.8 Conduct Disorder
       Specify type: Childhood-
       Onset Type/Adolescent-
       Onset Type
313.81 Oppositional Defiant
       Disorder
312.9 Disruptive Behavior Disorder
       NOS

**Feeding and Eating Disorders of
Infancy and Early Childhood**
307.52 Pica
307.53 Rumination Disorder
307.59 Feeding Disorder of Infancy
       or Early Childhood

Tic Disorders
307.23 Tourette's Disorder
307.22 Chronic Motor or Vocal Tic
       Disorder
307.21 Transient Tic Disorder
       Specify if: Single Episode/
       Recurrent
307.20 Tic Disorder NOS

Elimination Disorders
——.– Encopresis
787.6 With Constipation and
       Overflow Incontinence
307.7 Without Constipation and
       Overflow Incontinence
307.6 Enuresis (Not Due to a
       General Medical Condition)
       Specify type: Nocturnal
       Only/Diurnal Only/
       Nocturnal and Diurnal

**Other Disorders of Infancy,
Childhood, or Adolescence**
309.21 Separation Anxiety Disorder
       Specify if: Early Onset
313.23 Selective Mutism

313.89 Reactive Attachment
       Disorder of Infancy or Early
       Childhood
       Specify type: Inhibited Type/
       Disinhibited Type
307.3 Stereotypic Movement
       Disorder
       Specify if: With Self-Injurious
       Behavior
313.9 Disorder of Infancy,
       Childhood, or Adolescence
       NOS

**DELIRIUM, DEMENTIA,
AND AMNESTIC AND OTHER
COGNITIVE DISORDERS**

Delirium
293.0 Delirium Due to ... [Indicate
       the General Medical
       Condition]
——.– Substance Intoxication
       Delirium (refer to Sub-
       stance-Related Disorders for
       substance-specific codes)
——.– Substance Withdrawal
       Delirium (refer to Sub-
       stance-Related Disorders for
       substance-specific codes)
——.– Delirium Due to Multiple
       Etiologies (code each of the
       specific etiologies)
780.09 Delirium NOS

Dementia
290.xx Dementia of the Alzheimer's
       Type, With Early Onset
       (also code 331.0 Alzheimer's
       disease on Axis III)
  .10 Uncomplicated
  .11 With Delirium
  .12 With Delusions
  .13 With Depressed Mood

Specify if: With Behavioral Disturbance

290.xx Dementia of the Alzheimer's Type, With Late Onset (also code 331.0 Alzheimer's disease on Axis III)
.0 Uncomplicated
.3 With Delirium
.20 With Delusions
.21 With Depressed Mood
Specify if: With Behavioral Disturbance

290.xx Vascular Dementia
.40 Uncomplicated
.41 With Delirium
.42 With Delusions
.43 With Depressed Mood
Specify if: With Behavioral Disturbance

294.9 Dementia Due to HIV Disease (also code 043.1 HIV infection affecting central nervous system on Axis III)

294.1 Dementia Due to Head Trauma (also code 854.00 head injury on Axis III)

294.1 Dementia Due to Parkinson's disease (also code 332.0 Parkinson's disease on Axis III)

294.1 Dementia Due to Huntington's Disease (also code 333.4 Huntington's disease on Axis III)

290.10 Dementia Due to Pick's Disease (also code 331.1 Pick's disease on Axis III)

290.10 Dementia Due to Creutzfeldt-Jakob Disease (also code 046.1 Creutzfeldt-Jakob disease on Axis III)

294.1 Dementia Due to ... [Indicate the General Medical Condi-tion not listed above] (also code the general medical condition on Axis III)

—.– Substance-Induced Persisting Dementia (refer to Sub-stance-Related Disorders for substance-specific codes)

—.– Dementia Due to Multiple Etiologies (code each of the specific etiologies)

294.8 Dementia NOS

Amnestic Disorders

294.0 Amnestic Disorder Due to ... [Indicate the General Medi-cal Condition]
Specify if: Transient/Chronic

—.– Substance-Induced Persisting Amnestic Disorder (refer to Substance-Related Disorders for substance-specific codes)

294.8 Amnestic Disorder NOS

Other Cognitive Disorders

294.9 Cognitive Disorder NOS

MENTAL DISORDERS DUE TO A GENERAL MEDICAL CONDITION NOT ELSEWHERE CLASSIFIED

293.89 Catatonic Disorder Due to ... [Indicate the General Medical Condition]

310.1 Personality Change Due to ... [Indicate the General Medical Condition]
Specify type: Labile Type/Disinhibited Type/Aggres-sive Type/Apathetic Type/Paranoid Type/Other Type/Combined Type/Unspecified Type

293.9   Mental Disorder NOS Due to ... [Indicate the General Medical Condition]

SUBSTANCE-RELATED DISORDERS

[a]The following specifiers may be applied to Substance Dependence:
– With Physiological Dependence/ Without Physiological Dependence
– Early Full Remission/Early
– Partial Remission
– Sustained Full Remission/ Sustained Partial Remission
– On Agonist Therapy/In a Controlled Environment
   The following specifiers apply to Substance-Induced Disorders as noted:
– [I]With Onset During Intoxication/
[W]With Onset During Withdrawal

Alcohol-Related Disorders
Alcohol Use Disorders
303.90 Alcohol Dependence[a]
305.00 Alcohol Abuse
Alcohol-Induced Disorders
303.00 Alcohol Intoxication
291.8   Alcohol Withdrawal
        Specify if: With Perceptual Disturbances
291.0   Alcohol Intoxication Delirium
291.0   Alcohol Withdrawal Delirium
291.2   Alcohol-Induced Persisting Dementia
291.1   Alcohol-Induced Persisting Amnestic Disorder
291.x   Alcohol-Induced Psychotic Disorder
   .5   With Delusions[I,W]
   .3   With Hallucinations[I,W]
291.8   Alcohol-Induced Mood Disorder[I,W]

291.8   Alcohol-Induced Anxiety Disorder[I,W]
291.8   Alcohol-Induced Sexual Dysfunction[I]
291.8   Alcohol-Induced Sleep Disorder[I,W]
291.9   Alcohol-Related Disorder NOS

Amphetamine (or Amphetamine-like)-Related Disorders
Amphetamine Use Disorders
304.40 Amphetamine Dependence[a]
305.70 Amphetamine Abuse
Amphetamine-Induced Disorders
292.89 Amphetamine Intoxication
        Specify if: With Perceptual Disturbances
292.0   Amphetamine Withdrawal
292.81 Amphetamine Intoxication Delirium
292.xx Amphetamine-Induced Psychotic Disorder
   .11 With Delusions[I]
   .12 With Hallucinations[I]
292.84 Amphetamine-Induced Mood Disorder[I,W]
292.89 Amphetamine-Induced Anxiety Disorder[I]
292.89 Amphetamine-Induced Sexual Dysfunction[I]
292.89 Amphetamine-Induced Sleep Disorder[I,W]
292.9   Amphetamine-Related Disorder NOS

Caffeine-Related Disorders
Caffeine-Induced Disorders
305.90 Caffeine Intoxication
292.89 Caffeine-Induced Anxiety Disorder[I]
292.89 Caffeine-Induced Sleep Disorder[I]

292.9 Caffeine-Related Disorder
NOS

Cannabis-Related Disorders
Cannabis Use Disorders
304.30 Cannabis Dependence[a]
305.20 Cannabis Abuse
Cannabis-Induced Disorders
292.89 Cannabis Intoxication
Specify if: With Perceptual
Disturbances
292.81 Cannabis Intoxication
Delirium
292.xx Cannabis-Induced Psychotic
Disorder
.11 With Delusions[I]
.12 With Hallucinations[I]
292.89 Cannabis-Induced Anxiety
Disorder[I]
292.9 Cannabis-Related Disorder
NOS

Cocaine-Related Disorders
Cocaine Use Disorders
304.20 Cocaine Dependence[a]
305.60 Cocaine Abuse
Cocaine-Induced Disorders
292.89 Cocaine Intoxication
Specify if: With Perceptual
Disturbances
292.0 Cocaine Withdrawal
292.81 Cocaine Intoxication
Delirium
292.xx Cocaine-Induced Psychotic
Disorder
.11 With Delusions[I]
.12 With Hallucinations[I]
292.84 Cocaine-Induced Mood
Disorder[I,W]
292.89 Cocaine-Induced Anxiety
Disorder[I,W]
292.89 Cocaine-Induced Sexual
Dysfunction[I]

292.89 Cocaine-Induced Sleep
Disorder[I,W]
292.9 Cocaine-Related Disorder
NOS

Hallucinogen-Related Disorders
Hallucinogen Use Disorders
304.50 Hallucinogen Dependence[a]
305.30 Hallucinogen Abuse
Hallucinogen-Induced Disorders
292.89 Hallucinogen Intoxication
292.89 Hallucinogen Persisting
Perception Disorder (Flashbacks)
292.81 Hallucinogen Intoxication
Delirium
292.xx Hallucinogen-Induced
Psychotic Disorder
.11 With Delusions[I]
.12 With Hallucinations[I]
292.84 Hallucinogen-Induced Mood
Disorder[I]
292.89 Hallucinogen-Induced
Anxiety Disorder[I]
292.9 Hallucinogen-Related
Disorder NOS

Inhalant-Related Disorders
Inhalant Use Disorders
304.60 Inhalant Dependence[a]
305.90 Inhalant Abuse
Inhalant-Induced Disorders
292.89 Inhalant Intoxication
292.81 Inhalant Intoxication
Delirium
292.82 Inhalant-Induced Persisting
Dementia
292.xx Inhalant-Induced Psychotic
Disorder
.11 With Delusions[I]
.12 With Hallucinations[I]
292.84 Inhalant-Induced Mood
Disorder[I]

292.89 Inhalant-Induced Anxiety Disorder[I]
292.9 Inhalant-Related Disorder NOS

Nicotine-Related Disorders
Nicotine Use Disorder
305.10 Nicotine Dependence[a]
Nicotine-Induced Disorder
292.0 Nicotine Withdrawal
292.9 Nicotine-Related Disorder NOS

Opioid-Related Disorders
Opioid Use Disorders
304.00 Opioid Dependence[a]
305.50 Opioid Abuse
Opioid-Induced Disorders
292.89 Opioid Intoxication
Specify if: With Perceptual Disturbances
292.0 Opioid Withdrawal
292.81 Opioid Intoxication Delirium
292.xx Opioid-Induced Psychotic Disorder
.11 With Delusions[I]
.12 With Hallucinations[I]
292.84 Opioid-Induced Mood Disorder[I]
292.89 Opioid-Induced Sexual Dysfunction[I]
292.89 Opioid-Induced Sleep Disorder[I,W]
292.9 Opioid-Related Disorder NOS

Phencyclidine (or Phencyclidine-like)-Related Disorders
Phencyclidine Use Disorders
304.90 Phencyclidine Dependence[a]
305.90 Phencyclidine Abuse

Phencyclidine-Induced Disorders
292.89 Phencyclidine Intoxication
Specify if: With Perceptual Disturbances
292.81 Phencyclidine Intoxication Delirium
292.xx Phencyclidine-Induced Psychotic Disorder
.11 With Delusions[I]
.12 With Hallucinations[I]
292.84 Phencyclidine-Induced Mood Disorder[I]
292.89 Phencyclidine-Induced Anxiety Disorder[I]
292.9 Phencyclidine-Related Disorder NOS

Sedative-, Hypnotic-, or Anxiolytic-Related Disorders
Sedative, Hypnotic, or Anxiolytic Use Disorders
304.10 Sedative, Hypnotic, or Anxiolytic Dependence[a]
305.40 Sedative, Hypnotic, or Anxiolytic Abuse
Sedative-, Hypnotic-, or Anxiolytic-Induced Disorders
292.89 Sedative, Hypnotic, or Anxiolytic Intoxication
292.0 Sedative, Hypnotic, or Anxiolytic Withdrawal
Specify if: With Perceptual Disturbances
292.81 Sedative, Hypnotic, or Anxiolytic Intoxication Delirium
292.81 Sedative, Hypnotic, or Anxiolytic Withdrawal Delirium
292.82 Sedative-, Hypnotic-, or Anxiolytic-Induced Persisting Dementia

292.83 Sedative-, Hypnotic-, or Anxiolytic-Induced Persisting Amnestic Disorder

292.xx Sedative-, Hypnotic-, or Anxiolytic-Induced Psychotic Disorder
.11 With Delusions[I,W]
.12 With Hallucinations[I,W]

292.84 Sedative-, Hypnotic-, or Anxiolytic-Induced Mood Disorder[I,W]

292.89 Sedative-, Hypnotic-, or Anxiolytic-Induced Anxiety Disorder[W]

292.89 Sedative-, Hypnotic-, or Anxiolytic-Induced Sexual Dysfunction[I]

292.89 Sedative-, Hypnotic-, or Anxiolytic-Induced Sleep Disorder[I,W]

292.9 Sedative-, Hypnotic-, or Anxiolytic-Related Disorder NOS

Polysubstance-Related Disorder
304.80 Polysubstance Dependence[a]
Other (or Unknown) Substance-Related Disorders
Other (or Unknown) Substance Use Disorders
304.90 Other (or Unknown) Substance Dependence[a]
305.90 Other (or Unknown) Substance Abuse
Other (or Unknown) Substance-Induced Disorders
292.89 Other (or Unknown) Substance Intoxication
Specify if: With Perceptual Disturbances
292.0 Other (or Unknown) Substance Withdrawal
Specify if: With Perceptual Disturbances

292.81 Other (or Unknown) Substance-Induced Delirium

292.82 Other (or Unknown) Substance-Induced Persisting Dementia

292.83 Other (or Unknown) Substance-Induced Persisting Amnestic Disorder

292.xx Other (or Unknown) Substance-Induced Psychotic Disorder
.11 With Delusions[I,W]
.12 With Hallucinations[I,W]

292.84 Other (or Unknown) Substance-Induced Mood Disorder[I,W]

292.89 Other (or Unknown) Substance-Induced Anxiety Disorder[I,W]

292.89 Other (or Unknown) Substance-Induced Sexual Dysfunction[I]

292.89 Other (or Unknown) Substance-Induced Sleep Disorder[I,W]

292.9 Other (or Unknown) Substance-Related Disorder NOS

SCHIZOPHRENIA AND OTHER PSYCHOTIC DISORDERS

295.xx Schizophrenia
The following Classification of Longitudinal Course applies to all subtypes of Schizophrenia:
– Episodic With Interepisode Residual Symptoms (specify if: With Prominent Negative Symptoms)/
Episodic With No Interepisode Residual Symptoms/Continuous (specify if: With Prominent Negative Symptoms)

– Single Episode In Partial Remission (specify if: With Prominent Negative Symptoms)/Single Episode in Full Remission
–Other or Unspecified Pattern
  .30 Paranoid Type
  .10 Disorganized Type
  .20 Catatonic Type
  .90 Undifferentiated Type
  .60 Residual Type
295.40 Schizophreniform Disorder Specify if: Without Good Prognostic Features/With Good Prognostic Features
295.70 Schizoaffective Disorder Specify type: Bipolar Type/ Depressive Type
297.1 Delusional Disorder Specify type: Erotomanic Type/Grandiose Type/ Jealous Type/Persecutory Type/Somatic Type/Mixed Type/Unspecified Type
298.8 Brief Psychotic Disorder Specify if: With Marked Stressor(s)/Without Marked Stressor(s)/With Postpartum Onset
297.3 Shared Psychotic Disorder
293.xx Psychotic Disorder Due to ... [Indicate the General Medical Condition]
  .81 With Delusions
  .82 With Hallucinations
——.– Substance-Induced Psychotic Disorder (refer to Substance-Related Disorders for substance-specific codes) Specify if: With Onset During Intoxication/ With Onset During Withdrawal
298.9 Psychotic Disorder NOS

MOOD DISORDERS

Code current state of Major Depressive Disorder or Bipolar I Disorder in fifth digit:
1 = Mild
2 = Moderate
3 = Severe Without Psychotic Features
4 = Severe With Psychotic Features Specify: Mood-Congruent Psychotic Features/Mood-Incongruent Psychotic Features
5 = In Partial Remission
6 = In Full Remission
0 = Unspecified
  The following specifiers apply (for current or most recent episode) to Mood Disorders as noted:
– [a]Severity/Psychotic/Remission Specifiers/[b]Chronic/[c]With Catatonic Features/[d]With Melancholic Features/[e]With Atypical Features/ [f]With Postpartum Onset
  The following specifiers apply to Mood Disorders as noted:
– [g]With or Without Full interepisode Recovery/[h]With Seasonal Pattern/[i]With Rapid Cycling

Depressive Disorders
296.xx Major Depressive Disorder
  .2x Single Episode[a,b,c,d,e,f]
  .3x Recurrent[a,b,c,d,e,f,g,h]
300.4 Dysthymic Disorder Specify if: Early Onset/Late Onset Specify: With Atypical Features
311 Depressive Disorder NOS

Bipolar Disorders
296.xx Bipolar I Disorder
  .0x Single Manic Episod e[a,c,f] Specify if: Mixed

.40 Most Recent Episode Hypo-manic[g,h,i]

.4x Most Recent Episode Manic[a,c,f,g,h,i]

.6x Most Recent Episode Mixed[a,c,f,g,h,i]

.5x Most Recent Episode Depressed[a,b,c,d,e,f,g,h,i]

.7 Most Recent Episode Unspecified[g,h,i]

296.89 Bipolar II Disorder[a,b,c,d,e,f,g,h,i] Specify (current or most recent episode): Hypomanic/Depressed

301.13 Cyclothymic Disorder

296.80 Bipolar Disorder NOS

293.83 Mood Disorder Due to ... [Indicate the General Medical Condition] Specify type: With Depressive Features/With Major Depressive-Like Episode/ With Manic Features/With Mixed Features

——.– Substance-Induced Mood Disorder (refer to Substance-Related Disorders for substance-specific codes) Specify type: With Depressive Features/With Manic Features/With Mixed Features Specify if: With Onset During Intoxication/With Onset During Withdrawal

296.90 Mood Disorder NOS

ANXIETY DISORDERS

300.01 Panic Disorder Without Agoraphobia

300.21 Panic Disorder With Agoraphobia

300.22 Agoraphobia Without History of Panic Disorder

300.29 Specific Phobia Specify type: Animal Type/ Natural Environment Type/Blood-Injection-Injury Type/Situational Type/Other Type

300.23 Social Phobia Specify if: Generalized

300.3 Obsessive-Compulsive Disorder Specify if: With Poor Insight

309.81 Posttraumatic Stress Disorder Specify if: Acute/Chronic Specify if: With Delayed Onset

308.3 Acute Stress Disorder

300.02 Generalized Anxiety Disorder

293.89 Anxiety Disorder Due to ... [Indicate the General Medical Condition] Specify if: With Generalized Anxiety/With Panic Attacks/With Obsessive-Compulsive Symptoms

——.– Substance-Induced Anxiety Disorder (refer to Substance-Related Disorders for substance-specific codes) Specify if: With Generalized Anxiety/With Panic Attacks/ With Obsessive-Compulsive Symptoms/With Phobic Symptoms Specify if: With Onset During Intoxication/With Onset During Withdrawal

300.00 Anxiety Disorder NOS

SOMATOFORM DISORDERS

300.81 Somatization Disorder

300.81 Undifferentiated Somatoform Disorder

300.11 Conversion Disorder
Specify type: With Motor
Symptom or Deficit/With
Sensory Symptom or
Deficit/With Seizures or
Convulsions/With Mixed
Presentation
307.xx Pain Disorder
.80 Associated With
Psychological Factors
.89 Associated With Both
Psychological Factors and a
General Medical Condition
Specify if: Acute/ Chronic
300.7 Hypochondriasis
Specify if: With Poor Insight
300.7 Body Dysmorphic Disorder
300.81 Somatoform Disorder NOS

FACTITIOUS DISORDERS

300.xx Factitious Disorder
.16 With Predominantly
Psychological Signs and
Symptoms
.19 With Predominantly Physical
Signs and Symptoms
.19 With Combined
Psychological and Physical
Signs and Symptoms
300.19 Factitious Disorder NOS

DISSOCIATIVE DISORDERS

300.12 Dissociative Amnesia
300.13 Dissociative Fugue
300.14 Dissociative Identity Disorder
300.6 Depersonalization Disorder
300.15 Dissociative Disorder NOS

SEXUAL AND GENDER
IDENTITY DISORDERS

Sexual Dysfunctions
The following specifiers apply to all
primary Sexual Dysfunctions:
– Lifelong Type/ Acquired Type
– Generalized Type/ Situational Type
– Due to Psychological Factors/Due
   to Combined Factors

Sexual Desire Disorders
302.71 Hypoactive Sexual Desire
Disorder
302.79 Sexual Aversion Disorder

Sexual Arousal Disorders
302.72 Female Sexual Arousal
Disorder
302.72 Male Erectile Disorder

Orgasmic Disorders
302.73 Female Orgasmic Disorder
302.74 Male Orgasmic Disorder
302.75 Premature Ejaculation

Sexual Pain Disorders
302.76 Dyspareunia (Not Due to
General Medical Condition)
306.51 Vaginismus (Not Due to
General Medical Condition)

**Sexual Dysfunction Due to a
General Medical Condition**
625.8 Female Hypoactive Sexual
Desire Disorder Due to ...
[Indicate the General
Medical Condition]
608.89 Male Hypoactive Sexual
Desire Disorder Due to ...
[Indicate the General
Medical Condition]

607.84 Male Erectile Disorder Due to ... [Indicate the General Medical Condition]

625.0 Female Dyspareunia Due to ... [Indicate the General Medical Condition]

608.89 Male Dyspareunia Due to ... [Indicate the General Medical Condition]

625.8 Other Female Sexual Dysfunction Due to ... [Indicate the General Medical Condition]

608.89 Other Male Sexual Dysfunction Due to ... [Indicate the General Medical Condition]

——.– Substance-Induced Sexual Dysfunction (refer to Substance-Related Disorders for substance-specific codes) Specify if: With Impaired Desire/With Impaired Arousal/With Impaired Orgasm/With Sexual Pain Specify if: With Onset During Intoxication

302.70 Sexual Dysfunction NOS

Paraphilias

302.4 Exhibitionism

302.81 Fetishism

302.89 Frotteurism

302.2 Pedophilia Specify if: Sexually Attracted to Males/Sexually Attracted to Females/Sexually Attracted to Both Specify if: Limited to Incest Specify type: Exclusive Type/Nonexclusive Type

302.83 Sexual Masochism

302.84 Sexual Sadism

302.3 Transvestic Fetishism Specify if: With Gender Dysphoria

302.82 Voyeurism

302.9 Paraphilia NOS

Gender Identity Disorders

302.xx Gender Identity Disorder

.6 in Children

.85 in Adolescents or Adults Specify if: Sexually Attracted to Males/Sexually Attracted to Females/Sexually Attracted to Both/Sexually Attracted to Neither

302.6 Gender Identity Disorder NOS

302.9 Sexual Disorder NOS

EATING DISORDERS

307.1 Anorexia Nervosa Specify type: Restricting Type; Binge-Eating/Purging Type

307.51 Bulimia Nervosa Specify type: Purging Type/Nonpurging Type

307.50 Eating Disorder NOS

SLEEP DISORDERS

Primary Sleep Disorders

Dyssomnias

307.42 Primary Insomnia

307.44 Primary Hypersomnia Specify if: Recurrent

347 Narcolepsy

780.59 Breathing-Related Sleep Disorder

307.45 Circadian Rhythm Sleep Disorder Specify type: Delayed Sleep Phase Type/Jet Lag Type/Shift Work Type/Unspecified Type

307.47 Dyssomnia NOS
Parasomnias
307.47 Nightmare Disorder
307.46 Sleep Terror Disorder
307.46 Sleepwalking Disorder
307.47 Parasomnia NOS
Sleep Disorders Related to Another
    Mental Disorder
307.42 Insomnia Related to ...
    [Indicate the Axis I or Axis
    II Disorder]
307.44 Hypersomnia Related to ...
    [Indicate the Axis I or Axis
    II Disorder]

Other Sleep Disorders
780.xx Sleep Disorder Due to ...
    [Indicate the General
    Medical Condition]
  .52 Insomnia Type
  .54 Hypersomnia Type
  .59 Parasomnia Type
  .59 Mixed Type
——.– Substance-Induced Sleep
    Disorder (refer to Substance-
    Related Disorders for
    substance-specific codes)
    Specify type: Insomnia Type/
    Hypersomnia Type/
    Parasomnia Type/Mixed
    Type
    Specify if: With Onset
    During Intoxication/ With
    Onset During Withdrawal

IMPULSE-CONTROL DISORDERS NOT ELSEWHERE CLASSIFIED

312.34 Intermittent Explosive
    Disorder
312.32 Kleptomania
312.33 Pyromania
312.31 Pathological Gambling

312.39 Trichotillomania
312.30 Impulse-Control Disorder
    NOS

ADJUSTMENT DISORDERS

309.xx Adjustment Disorder
  .0 With Depressed Mood
  .24 With Anxiety
  .28 With Mixed Anxiety and De-
    pressed Mood
  .3 With Disturbance of Conduct
  .4 With Mixed Disturbance of
    Emotions and Conduct Un-
    specified
  .9 Unspecified
    Specify if: Acute/Chronic

PERSONALITY DISORDERS

Note: These are coded on Axis II.
301.0 Paranoid Personality Disorder
301.20 Schizoid Personality Disorder
301.22 Schizotypal Personality
    Disorder
301.7 Antisocial Personality Disorder
301.83 Borderline Personality
    Disorder
301.50 Histrionic Personality
    Disorder
301.81 Narcissistic Personality
    Disorder
301.82 Avoidant Personality Disorder
301.6 Dependent Personality
    Disorder
301.4 Obsessive-Compulsive
    Personality Disorder
301.9 Personality Disorder NOS

OTHER CONDITIONS
THAT MAY BE A FOCUS OF
CLINICAL ATTENTION

Psychological Factors Affecting Medical Condition
316　... [Specified Psychological Factor] Affecting ... [Indicate the General Medical Condition]
Choose name based on nature of factors:
Mental Disorder Affecting Medical Condition
Psychological Symptoms Affecting Medical Condition
Personality Traits or Coping Style Affecting Medical Condition
Maladaptive Health Behaviors Affecting Medical Condition
Stress-Related Physiological Response Affecting Medical Condition
Other or Unspecified Psychological Factors Affecting Medical Condition

Medication-Induced Movement Disorders
332.1　Neuroleptic-Induced Parkinsonism
333.92　Neuroleptic Malignant Syndrome
333.7　Neuroleptic-Induced Acute Dystonia
333.99　Neuroleptic-Induced Acute Akathisia
333.82　Neuroleptic-Induced Tardive Dyskinesia
333.1　Medication-Induced Postural Tremor
333.90　Medication-Induced Movement Disorder NOS

Other Medication-Induced Disorder
995.2　Adverse Effects of Medication NOS

Relational Problems
V61.9　Relational Problem Related to a Mental Disorder or General Medical Condition
V61.20　Parent-Child Relational Problem
V61.1　Partner Relational Problem
V61.8　Sibling Relational Problem
V62.81　Relational Problem NOS

Problems Related to Abuse or Neglect
V61.21　Physical Abuse of Child (code 995.5 if focus of attention is on victim)
V61.21　Sexual Abuse of Child (code 995.5 if focus of attention is on victim)
V61.21　Neglect of Child (code 995.5 if focus of attention is on victim)
V61.1　Physical Abuse of Adult (code 995.81 if focus of attention is on victim)
V61.1　Sexual Abuse of Adult (code 995.81 if focus of attention is on victim)

Additional Conditions That May Be a Focus of Clinical Attention
V15.81　Noncompliance with Treatment
V65.2　Malingering
V71.01　Adult Antisocial Behavior
V71.02　Child or Adolescent Antisocial Behavior
V62.89　Borderline Intellectual Functioning
Note: This is coded on Axis II.

780.9   Age-Related Cognitive Decline
V62.82 Bereavement
V62.3   Academic Problem
V62.2   Occupational Problem
313.82 Identity Problem
V62.89 Religious or Spiritual
        Problem
V62.4   Acculturation Problem
V62.89 Phase of Life Problem

ADDITIONAL CODES

300.9   Unspecificied Mental Disorder
        (nonpsychotic)
V71.09 No Diagnosis or Condition
        on Axis I
799.9   Diagnosis or Condition
        Deferred on Axis I
V71.09 No Diagnosis on Axis II
799.9   Diagnosis Deferred on Axis II

MULTIAXIAL SYSTEM

Axis I   Clinical Disorders
        Other Conditions That May
        Be a Focus of Clinical
        Attention
Axis II Personality Disorders
        Mental Retardation
Axis III General Medical Conditions
Axis IV Psychosocial and Environ-
        mental Problems
Axis V Global Assessment of
        Functioning

Used with permission. *Diagnostic and Statistical Manual of Mental Disorders,* 4th ed. Washington, D.C.: American Psychiatric Association, 1994.

Sexual and Sleep Disorders

◆ I. Sexual and gender identity disorders
A. Related *DSM-IV* medical diagnoses
1. Sexual dysfunctions
   a. Sexual desire disorders
      (1) Hypoactive sexual desire disorder
      (2) Sexual aversion disorder
   b. Sexual arousal disorders
      (1) Female sexual arousal disorder
      (2) Male erectile disorder
   c. Orgasmic disorders
      (1) Female orgasmic disorder
      (2) Male orgasmic disorder
      (3) Premature ejaculation
   d. Sexual pain disorders
      (1) Dyspareunia (not due to a general medical condition)
      (2) Vaginismus (not due to a general medical condition)
   e. Sexual dysfunction due to a general medical condition
2. Paraphilias
   a. Exhibitionism
   b. Fetishism
   c. Frotteurism
   d. Pedophilia
   e. Sexual masochism
   f. Sexual sadism
   g. Transvestic fetishism
   h. Voyeurism
   i. Paraphilia NOS
3. Gender identity disorders
   a. Gender identity disorder in children, adolescents, adults
   b. Gender identity disorder NOS
   c. Sexual disorder NOS

B. Related NANDA nursing diagnoses
1. Anxiety
2. Ineffective individual coping
3. Disturbed body image
4. Knowledge deficit
5. Pain

6. Altered role performance
7. Sexual dysfunction
8. Altered sexuality patterns
9. Social isolation

◆ II. Sleep disorders

A. Related *DSM-IV* medical diagnoses
   1. Primary sleep disorders
      a. Dyssomnias
         (1) Primary insomnia
         (2) Primary hypersomnia
         (3) Narcolepsy
         (4) Breathing-related sleep disorder
         (5) Circadium rhythm sleep disorder
         (6) Dyssomnia NOS
      b. Parasomnias
         (1) Nightmare disorder
         (2) Sleep terror disorder
         (3) Sleepwalking disorder
         (4) Parasomnia NOS
   2. Sleep disorders related to another mental disorder
      a. Insomnia related to (specify)
      b. Hypersomnia related to (specify)
   3. Other sleep disorders
      a. Sleep disorder related to (specify)
      b. Substance-induced sleep disorder

B. Related NANDA nursing diagnoses
   1. Anxiety
   2. Ineffective individual coping
   3. Fatigue
   4. Altered health-maintenance
   5. Disturbed sleep pattern

Selected References

Anai-Otong, D. *Psychiatric Nursing: Biological and Behavioral Concepts.* Philadelphia: W.B. Saunders Co., 1995.

Brackley, M.H. *Instructor's Manual for Psychiatric Nursing: Biological and Behavioral Concepts.* Philadelphia: W.B. Saunders Co., 1995.

Burgess, A.W. *Psychiatric Nursing in the Hospital and Community,* 5th ed. Norwalk, Conn.: Appleton & Lange, 1990.

Fontaine, K.L., and Fletcher, J.S. *Essentials of Mental Health Nursing,* 3rd ed. Redwood City, Calif.: Addison-Wesley, 1995.

Johnson, B. S. *Psychiatric Mental Health Nursing Adaptation and Growth,* 3rd ed. Philadelphia: J.B. Lippincott Co., 1993.

Krupnick, S.L.W., and Wade, A.J. *Psychiatric Care Planning.* Springhouse, Pa.: Springhouse Corporation, 1993.

Gary, F., and Kavanagh, C.K. *Psychiatric Mental Health Nursing.* Philadelphia: J.B. Lippincott Co., 1991.

McFarland, G.K., and Thomas, M.D. *Psychiatric Mental Health Nursing: Application of the Nursing Process.* Philadelphia: J.B. Lippincott Co., 1991.

Schultz, J.M., and Videbeck, S.D. *Manual of Psychiatric Care Plans,* 4th ed. Philadelphia: J.B. Lippincott Co., 1994.

Stuart, G.W., and Sundeen, S.J. *Principles and Practice of Psychiatric Nursing,* 5th ed. St. Louis: Mosby–Year Book, Inc., 1995.

Index

A

Adaptive social responses
    characteristics of, 101
    development of, throughout life
        cycle, 101-102
Addiction, 109, 161
Affect, 68, 92, 161
Aggression, 161
    behavioral cues for, 129
    characteristics of, 127
    cognitive cues for, 130
    diagnoses related to, 130
    nursing interventions for, 130-131
    patient outcomes for, 130
    precipitating stressors in, 128
    teaching plan for, 129
    theories of, 127-128
    treatment modalities for, 128-130
Aggression-turned-inward theory, 69
Alcohol abuse, 112. *See also* Substance
    abuse.
    diagnoses related to, 114
    nursing interventions for, 114-115
    phases of, 112-113
    physiologic consequences of, 113
    withdrawal behavior and, 113
Alexithymia, 161
Alienation, 161
Alzheimer's disease, 161. *See also*
    Dementia.
    teaching plan for, 146
Ambivalence, 92
American Nurses Association (ANA)
    certification by, 3
    practice standards of, 3, 7-8
Amnesia, 52
Anger
    characteristics of, 124
    dysfunctional, 124
    expressions of, 124-125
    functional, 124
    nursing interventions for, 126-127
    patient outcomes for, 126

Anger *(continued)*
    responses associated with, 125-126
Anhedonia, 161
Anorexia nervosa, 156. *See also* Eating
    disorders.
Anticipatory guidance, 161
Antidepressants, 71
Antimanic medications, 71
Anxiety
    affective responses to, 58
    behavioral responses to, 58
    characteristics of, 56
    cognitive responses to, 58
    coping strategies for, 58-59
    diagnoses related to, 59
    levels of, 56-57
    nursing interventions for, 59-60
    origins of, 56
    patient outcomes for, 59
    physiologic responses to, 57-58
    precipitating stressors in, 57
Anxiety disorders
    characteristics of, 60
    diagnoses related to, 60-61
    nursing interventions for, 61
    patient outcomes for, 61
    types of, 61-65
Anxiety disorders of childhood, 154
    diagnoses related to, 155
    nursing interventions for, 155
    patient outcomes for, 155
    types of, 154-155
Associative looseness, 91-92
Attention deficit hyperactive disorder,
    151-152. *See also* Disruptive be-
    havior disorders.
Attention deficit without hyperactivity
    disorder, 152. *See also* Disruptive
    behavior disorders.
Attitudinal restructuring, 161
Autistic disorder, 150
    assessment of, 150
    diagnoses related to, 150-151
    nursing interventions for, 151

i refers to an illustration; t refers to a table.

Autistic disorder *(continued)*
    patient outcomes for, 151
Autistic thinking, 92, 161
Autogenic training, 161
Automatism, 161
Avoidance, 111

B
Beck, Aaron, 16, 17, 70
Behavioral model, 12, 70
Behavior modification, 161
Binge eating, 161. *See also* Bulimia nervosa.
Biofeedback, 161
Biogenic model, 20
Biological therapies, 30
Bipolar disorder, 68
Body image, 48, 161
    alterations in, 93-94
Bowlby, J., 70
Brain abnormalities, schizophrenia and, 89
Bulimia nervosa, 157. *See also* Eating disorders.

C
Caplan, Gerald, 17
Carbamazepine, 71
Certification, 3, 6
Child abuse, 135, 137
Circadian rhythms, mood disorders and, 69
Clang association, 93, 161
Cocaine intoxication, immediate care for, 119i
Cognitive behavioral therapy, 29-30
Cognitive development, stages of, 16
Cognitive model, 16-17, 70
Cognitive therapy, 162
Cognitive triad, 17
Community mental health, 2, 17, 162
Community Mental Health Act (1963), 2
Conceptual models, 11-22
Conduct disorder, 152. *See also* Disruptive behavior disorders.
Confabulation, 162
Consensual validation, 162
Conversion disorder, 162
Coping mechanisms, 162

Counter-conditioning, 162
Crisis intervention, 24-25, 162

D
Death
    assessment of, 40
    coping stages of, 40
    diagnoses related to, 41
    emotional responses to, 40
    nursing interventions for, 41
    patient outcomes for, 41
    teaching plan for, 42
Defense mechanisms, 162
Degenerative dementia, 162
Delayed grief reactions, 43, 44
Delirium, 142
    characteristics of, 142-143
    diagnoses related to, 143
    nursing interventions for, 143
    patient outcomes for, 143
Delusions, 93, 96-97
Dementia, 143-144
    characteristics of, 144-145
    diagnoses related to, 145
    nursing interventions for, 145-146
    patient outcomes for, 145
Dependency, 103-104
Depersonalization, 50, 162
Depersonalization disorders, 52
Depressant abuse, 111, 117
Depression, 68, 69, 72-76, 74i, 75t, 82
Desensitization, 162
Designer drugs, 111
Development
    schizophrenia and, 90
    stages of, 15t
Developmental model, 14-15
Diagnostic and Statistical Manual of Mental Disorders, Fourth Edition, Revised (DSM-IV), classifications in, 13, 179-192
Dichotomous thinking, 162
Disruptive behavior disorders
    diagnoses related to, 153
    nursing interventions for, 153
    patient outcomes for, 153
    types of, 151-153
Dissociative disorders, 52
Distorted grief reactions, 43, 44
Drug abuse, 115. *See also* Substance abuse.
    diagnoses related to, 118

i refers to an illustration; t refers to a table.

Drug abuse *(continued)*
  manifestations of, 116-117
  nursing interventions for, 118-120
  physiologic consequences
    of, 115-116

E

Eating disorders, 155
  diagnoses related to, 157-158
  nursing interventions for, 158-159
  patient outcomes for, 158
  teaching plan for, 158
  types of, 156-157
Echolalia, 93, 162
Ectomorph, 20
Ego boundaries, establishing, 96
Ego-dystonic behaviors, 163
Ego identity, 48
Ego-syntonic behaviors, 163
Elder abuse, 135, 137
Electroconvulsive therapy, 71
Ellis, Albert, 12
Empathy, 163
Encounter group therapy, 163
Endocrine dysfunction, mood disorders
    and, 69
Endomorph, 20
Erikson, Erik, 14, 15t
Exhibitionism, 163
Existentialism, 163
Existential model, 12-13

F

Family therapy, 28
Family violence and abuse
  categories of, 134-135
  causes of, 135
  characteristics of family system in, 136
  characteristics of offenders in, 136-137
  characteristics of victims in, 137-138
  diagnoses related to, 138
  epidemiology of, 135
  nursing interventions for, 138-139
  patient outcomes for, 138
  theories of, 134
  treatment modalities for, 136
Fear, 163
Feedback, 163
Flight-or-fight response, 18t, 163
Free association, 163
Freud, Anna, 14

Freud, Sigmund, 13, 69
Fromm-Reichman, Freida, 14
Fugue, 52

G

Gender identity disorders, 193-194
General adaptation syndrome, stages
    of, 18t
Generalized anxiety disorder in child-
    hood, 154. *See also* Anxiety disor-
    ders of childhood.
Generalized anxiety state, 61. *See also*
    Anxiety disorders.
  characteristics of, 61-62
  nursing interventions for, 62
Genetic transmission
  bipolar disorder and, 68
  schizophrenia and, 89
Gestalt therapy, 163
Glasser, William, 12
Grandiosity, 111
Grieving, 42
  assessment of, 43
  diagnoses related to, 43-44
  manifestations of, 43
  nursing interventions for, 44
  patient outcomes for, 44
  types of, 42-43
Group therapy, 26-28
Guided imagery, 163

H

Hallucinations, 93, 97, 163
Hallucinogen abuse, 117
Healthy personality, characteristics of, 49
Heidegger, Martin, 12
Helplessness, 103-104
  learned, 70
Holistic, 163
Horney, Karen, 14
Hostility, 163
Hydrotherapy, 163
Hyperonality, 163
Hypnosis, 163
Hypochondriasis, 94, 163

I

Id, 163
Identity, 48, 164
  confusion associated with, 49-50, 94
Impulsivity, 105-106, 111
Incest, 164

Inhalant abuse, 111, 117
Interpersonal development, phases of, 16
Interpersonal model, 15-16

JKL
Jung, Carl, 14
Kierkegaard, Soren, 12
King, I., 19
Klein, Melanie, 14
Laing, R.D., 12
Learned helplessness, 70
Lethality, 164
Lewinsohn, P., 70
Lithium, 71-72

M
Magical thinking, 164
Mania, 68, 69, 76-78
Manipulation, 105-106, 110
Marijuana abuse, 117
Medical model, 13
Menninger, Karl, 14
Mental health nursing. *See* Psychiatric
    nursing.
Mental Health Survey Act (1955), 2
Mental Health Systems Act (1981), 3
Mental retardation
    assessment of, 149
    classification of, 149
    diagnoses related to, 149
    nursing interventions for, 150
    patient outcomes for, 149
Milieu, 164
Milieu therapy, 2, 164
Modeling, 164
Models, conceptual, 11-22
    behavioral, 12
    biogenic, 20
    cognitive, 16-17
    developmental, 14-15
    existential, 12-13
    interpersonal, 15-16
    medical, 13
    nursing, 19
    psychoanalytic, 13-14
    social, 17
    stress-adaptation, 17-19
Mood disorders, 68
    classification of, 68
    depressive reactions in, 72-76
    diagnoses related to, 72

Mood disorders *(continued)*
    epidemioloy of, 70
    etiology of, 68-70
    manic reactions in, 76-78
    treatments for, 71-72
Mutism, 93, 164

N
Narcotherapy, 164
National Institute of Mental Health
    (NIMH), 2, 3
National Mental Health Act (1946), 2
Neglect, 135
Neologism, 93, 164
Neurotic behavior, 164
Neurotransmitter, 164
Neurotransmitter imbalance
    mood disorders and, 68-69
    schizophrenia and, 90
North American Nursing Diagnosis As-
    sociation (NANDA) taxonomy,
    176-178
Nurse generalist, 6
Nurse practice acts, performance level
    and, 5
Nurse specialist, 6
Nursing model, 19

O
Object-loss theory, 70
Obsessive-compulsive disorder, 63. *See
    also* Anxiety disorders.
    characteristics of, 63
    nursing interventions for, 63-64
Obsessive-compulsive disorder of child-
    hood, 155. *See also* Anxiety disor-
    ders of childhood.
Operant conditioning, 164
Opiate abuse, 111, 116
Oppositional defiant disorder, 152-153.
    See also Disruptive behavior
    disorders.
Orem, D., 19

PQ
Paraphilias, 193
Pavlov, Ivan, 12
Peplau, H., 19
Perception, 164
Perls, Frederick, 12
Personality disorders
    characteristics of, 102

i refers to an illustration; t refers to a table.

Personality disorders *(continued)*
  predisposing factors in, 102-103
  teaching plan for, 103
  treatment modalities for, 103
Phobias, 62. *See also* Anxiety disorders.
  characteristics of, 62-63
  nursing interventions for, 63
  teaching plan for, 63
Phototherapy, 72, 164
Physical abuse, 134-135
Physical dependence, 109
Piaget, Jean, 16
Post-traumatic stress disorder, 64. *See also* Anxiety disorders.
  characteristics of, 64
  nursing interventions for, 64
Primary prevention, 164
Projection, 164
Psychiatric nursing
  ANA practice standards for, 7-9
  factors determining performance level of, 5-6
  history of, 2-3
  practice settings for, 5
  roles and functions of, 3-5
Psychoanalytic model, 13-14
Psychodrama, 164
Psychogenic fugue, 164
Psychogenic pain, 164
Psychological autopsy, 164
Psychological dependence, 165
Psychological unavailability, 135
Psychosexual development, stages of, 14
Psychosis, 165
Psychosurgery, 165
Psychotherapy, individual, 28-29
Psychotic behavior, 89, 165
Purge, 165. *See also* Bulimia nervosa.

R

Rape trauma
  characteristics of, 131, 132-133
  diagnoses related to, 133
  incidence of, 131
  motivations for attack in, 132
  nursing interventions for, 133-134
  patient outcomes for, 133
  treatment modalities for, 132
  victim's reactions and, 132
Rapid eye movement, depression and, 69
Rational-emotive therapy, 165

Reaction formation, 165
Reality therapy, 165
Relationship therapy, 165
Resistance, 165
Robertson, J., 70
Rogers, Carl, 12
Rogers, M., 19
Role clarification, 165
Role modeling, 165
Role playing, 165
Role reversal, 165
Roy, C., 19
Rumination, 165

S

Sartre, Jean Paul, 12
Schizoaffective disorder, 165
Schizophrenia, 82, 89
  affect and, 92
  body image alterations and, 93-94
  causative theories of, 89-90
  diagnoses related to, 94-95
  manifestations of, 91-94
  nursing interventions for, 95-97
  patient outcomes for, 95
  steps in process of, 90
  teaching plan for, 92
  treatment modalities for, 91
  types of, 90-91
School phobia disorder, 154. *See also* Anxiety disorders of childhood.
Seasonal affective disorder, 72, 165
Seasonal variations, mood disorders and, 69, 72
Seclusion, 165
Secondary prevention, 165
Selective inattention, 166
Self-actualization, 166
Self-awareness, 12, 166
Self-concept, 48, 166
  alterations in
    behaviors associated with, 49-50
    diagnoses related to, 50
    nursing interventions for, 51-52
    patient outcomes for, 50
    teaching plan for, 51
  components of, 48-49
  healthy personality and, 49
Self-destructive behavior, 166
Self-esteem, 49, 166
Self-ideals, 49
Seligman, Martin, 70

Selye, Hans, 17
Semantic fallacies, 166
Separation anxiety disorder, 154. *See also*
    Anxiety disorders of childhood.
Sexual abuse, 135
Sexual assault. *See* Rape trauma.
Sexual disorders, 193-194
Sexual dysfunctions, 193
Skinner, B.F., 12
Sleep disorders, 194
Sleep manipulation, 72
Social model, 17
Somatic therapies, 166
Somatoform disorders, 64. *See also*
    Anxiety disorders.
    characteristics of, 64-65
    nursing interventions for, 65
Spitz, R., 70
Spouse abuse, 135, 137
Stimulant abuse, 111, 116-117
Stress
    adaptation to, 18-19, 34
    assessment of, 35-36
    diagnoses related to, 36
    illness related to, 34-35
    management strategies for, 36-37
    nursing interventions for, 36
    patient outcomes for, 36
    physiological responses to, 18t, 34, 35
    symptoms of, 34
    teaching plan for, 37
Stress-adaptation model, 17-19
Stressors, 34, 70, 166
Substance abuse, 82, 109. *See also* Alco-
    hol abuse *and* Drug abuse.
    behaviors associated with, 110-111
    common drugs used in, 111
    patterns of, 109
    predisposing factors in, 110
    prevalence of, 110
    teaching plan for, 120
    treatment modalities for, 112
Substance dependence, 109
Suicidal behavior, 81
    diagnoses related to, 84
    epidemiology of, 81
    manifestations of, 83-84
    myths about, 81
    nursing interventions for, 84-86
    patient outcomes for, 84
    risk factors in, 82-83

Suicidal behavior *(continued)*
    teaching plan for, 86
    theories of, 81-82
    treatment modalities for, 84
Suicide, 166
Suicide ideation, 166
Sullivan, Harry Stack, 2, 15
Superego, 166
Supportive confrontation, 166
Suspiciousness, 104-105
Symbolization, 166
Szasz, Thomas, 17

T
Tangentiality, 93, 166
Tertiary prevention, 166
Therapeutic environment, 25-26
Therapeutic touch, 166
Token economy system, 166
Tolerance, physical dependence
    and, 109, 166
Transference, 167
Transmethylation, 167
Treatment modalities, 24-32

U
Uncomplicated grief reaction, 167
Undoing, 167

V
Valproic acid, 72
Verbal hostility, 135
Violence, 167. *See also* Aggression.
Visualization, 167

WXYZ
Watson, 19
Withdrawal, 105, 109, 113
Withdrawal syndrome, 167
Wolpe, J., 12
Word salad, 93, 167

i refers to an illustration; t refers to a table.

About the
StudySmart Disk

StudySmart Disk lets you:
- review subject areas of your choice and learn the rationales for the correct answers
- take tests of varying lengths on subjects of your choice
- print the results of your tests to gauge your progress over time.

Recommended system requirements
486 IBM-compatible personal computer (386 minimum)
Windows 3.1 or greater (Windows 95 compatible)
High-density 3½" floppy drive
8 MB RAM (4 MB minimum)
S-VGA monitor (VGA minimum)
2 MB of available space on hard drive

Installing and running the program
- Start Windows.
- In Program Manager, choose Run from File menu.
- Insert disk, type a:\setup.exe (where a: is the letter of your floppy drive), and click on OK.

For Windows 95 Installation
- Start Windows.
- Select Start button and then Run.
- Insert disk, type a:\setup.exe (where a: is the letter of your floppy drive), and click on OK.

For technical support, call 215-628-7744 Monday through Friday, 9 a.m. to 6 p.m. Eastern Standard Time.

The clinical information and tools in the *StudySmart Disk* are based on research and consultation with nursing, medical, and legal authorities. To the best of our knowledge, this program reflects currently accepted practice; nevertheless, it can't be considered absolute or universal. For individual application, all recommendations must be considered in light of the patient's clinical condition and, before administration of new or infrequently used drugs, in light of the latest package-insert information. The authors and publisher disclaim responsibility for any adverse effects resulting directly or indirectly from the suggested procedures, from any undetected errors, or from the reader's misunderstanding of the program.

This book cannot be returned for credit or refund if the vinyl disk holder has been opened, broken, or otherwise tampered with.